Praise for *A Modern Approach to the Birds and the Bees*

"*A Modern Approach to the Birds and the Bees* is the only book you'll need for teaching sex education. It is a clear, comprehensive, modern guidebook for all things related to sexuality. Every parent needs this book right next to their copy of *What to Expect When You're Expecting* on their bookshelf. It is a resource they'll grab again and again throughout their children's lives. Every teacher needs this as a reference book as well. I only wish I'd had this book sooner."

—Amanda DeLis-Mireles, mother of four (ages four to seventeen) and teacher

"*A Modern Approach to the Birds and the Bees* is a tremendous resource for parents! My sons are in first and seventh grade, and the book eased my anxiety around sexual education by providing age-appropriate information and discussions ideas. It is not too early to protect and prepare my sons for healthy sexuality, and I am now armed to do so."

—Tena Merkel Baker, parent

"As both a new step-mom and a woman who grew up with internet access before it was as monitored as it is now, I find this book an enlightening and informative resource to have, not only for navigating these conversations with my own kids, but for undoing two decades of misinformation and misunderstanding of my own sexuality and sexual health. Robin's book bridges the gap between generations who have had no real acceptance and understanding of sexual health and education, and a younger generation who is bombarded with unfiltered, often unsolicited, information regarding their own sexuality."

—Kaylee Goins

"Dr. Pickering brings a balanced, factual perspective into an arena that is presently governed by shame and confusion. In current sexual education models, there is a vast gap between what is evidence-based and what is in current practice. Dr. Pickering fills this gap with information and practical tools, making this book applicable for healthcare workers, parents, or anyone looking to understand the current sexual landscape of our culture. She has drawn from a wide variety of resources to compile a comprehensive guide that outlines the 'what' and the 'how' to talk to children and young adults about sexual health and relationships with confidence and clarity. I hope that this resource will empower parents and healthcare workers to support children through life's transitions to become emotionally and physically healthy adults."

—Allison Grefsrud, BA Health Science and student of
Naturopathic Medicine

"As a mom of two young adult men, I truly enjoyed reading this book and only wish I could've read it earlier, when we first started talking about sex in our house. Perhaps the biggest benefits here are her real-world guides to navigating discussions about consent and breakups, the points where a compassionate parent needs guidance to discuss relationship topics normally only broached within a friendship circle. I recommend this book for all parents looking to connect with their maturing kids and help with relationship development."

—Amy Biviano, MBA, CPA

A Modern Approach to

the Birds

& the Bees

A Modern Approach to
the Birds
& the Bees

A Parent's Comprehensive Guide to Talking about Sexuality

Robin Pickering, PhD

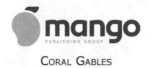

CORAL GABLES

A Modern Approach to the Birds and the Bees: A Parent's Comprehensive
Guide to Talking about Sexuality

Library of Congress Cataloging-in-Publication number: 2020940934
ISBN: (print) 978-1-64250-325-8, (ebook) 978-1-64250-326-5
BISAC category code: FAM034000, FAMILY & RELATIONSHIPS / Parenting
/ General

Printed in the United States of America

Table of Contents

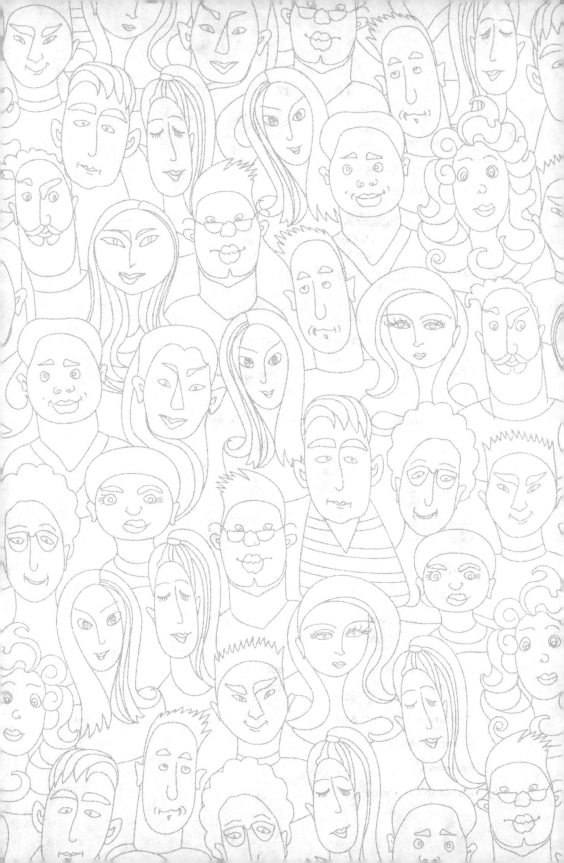

Introduction

When my daughter first asked how babies were made, she was six years old and, like most kids her age, very inquisitive. I was in graduate school, fully engulfed in my studies which included advanced coursework in human sexuality and health education. I found myself particularly interested in the concept of "age appropriate" sexuality education, as it was so different from what was actually being taught in schools and by even the brightest parents that I knew. The more I learned about anatomy and physiology and reproduction and sexually transmitted infections, the larger the gap appeared between science and practice.

So when my daughter approached me with her question, I was ecstatic! Unlike many of my friends, I was looking forward to launching into the next phase of our mother/daughter relationship. It felt as though the time and money I had invested in grad school were about to come to fruition, and I was anxious to apply what I had learned and practice my newly acquired teaching skills.

I took a breath, and with great pride launched into my monologue. She listened intently and with great interest to my carefully delivered speech.

And then, silence.

A curious look.

Silence.

A disturbed look.

And then more silence.

When she was finally ready to speak, she looked me in the eye and matter-of-factly stated, "Well, that's the grossest thing I have ever heard, and I wish you would have never told me." I let out a laugh, and we didn't resume the conversation for at least another year.

I often think about that story when I reflect on my passion for educating kids and parents about sexuality. Even as a person who has taken many doctorate-level courses on education and sexuality and has taught in that area for many years, I find that parental discussions about issues concerning sexuality can be difficult. Really difficult. And although talking to kids about sex has never been an easy task, it seems that a variety of factors make those discussions even more difficult in a modern context. With this book, my hope is that those discussions will be a little easier and a lot more effective.

Talking about Sex in a Modern Context Is Necessary but Difficult

Unquestionably, a changing social and technological environment brings new concerns for parents. Changing attitudes toward sexuality, the pervasiveness of internet access and social media, "sexting," and new legal and social standards around issues of consent raise understandable anxiety and uncertainty for parents who may ask themselves questions such as:

- How do I talk to my kids about my expectations concerning sexuality?

- How do I keep them safe from online predators?

- How do I teach them about personal boundaries?

- How do I navigate conversations around gender identity and same-sex behavior?

- How do I effectively encourage abstinence and discuss ways to avoid sexually transmitted infections and unwanted pregnancies?

- How do I teach about consent in a post #MeToo society in order to prepare my children for their futures as successful adults?

- How do I provide an alternative to the information that they are bombarded with in movies and music and social media?

- What are they teaching my kids at school and what am I supposed to be teaching at home?

There has been great debate about the delivery of sexuality education, with many expressing passionately that it should happen in schools and a vocal minority just as passionately stating that home is the place where those conversations should occur. Although there is disagreement concerning *where* sexuality education should occur and *what content* is appropriate, most parents agree that educating children about sexuality is important, and they demonstrate a desire to raise healthy children who will later mature to be sexually healthy adults. And while some parents may be comfortable talking about fairly straightforward topics like puberty or abstinence, many find themselves ill-equipped to tackle more complex issues that are necessary to give children and young adults the tools they need to navigate the complex challenges that they will encounter in a modern context.

Though it may often feel like children aren't listening or, like my daughter, think "it's the grossest thing they've ever heard," parental conversations about sex matter. Research indicates that young people whose parents effectively communicated with them about sex are *more likely to delay sex, have fewer partners, and use contraception if they do have sex.* There is also significant data to suggest that in countries where children are exposed to a more comprehensive sexuality education, rates of teen pregnancies are significantly lower than in countries where education is abstinence-only based and revolves around dangers and cautionary tales.

Many parents want to communicate with their children about issues related to sex, but they often simply lack the information to effectively do so. Modern methods of birth control, increased exposure to sexually explicit content, and changing norms around sexual behavior can make parents feel "out of touch" with issues that young people face and unsure of where to go to find accurate information.

School Sex Ed: Benefits and Limitations

Accurate sexuality education can protect children from exploitive or risky activities that may lead to unintended pregnancy, health and social problems, unnecessary risk of sexual assault, and sexually transmitted infections. Children receive information about sexuality from a variety of sources, and, when their questions go unanswered, they will often turn to less than ideal "experts" to get information. Effective school sexuality education coupled with informed parental conversations can be an important part of supporting positive outcomes.

In order to understand how to effectively tackle complex issues like teen pregnancy, sexually transmitted infections, and sexual assault, it makes sense to look at successful models of school sexuality education which we can emulate. Fortunately, there are many examples of effective approaches from which we can draw.

According to the Guttmacher Institute, European countries tend to have the lowest rates of teen pregnancy. Italy, Germany, and Switzerland, among others, had fewer than four teen births per thousand babies born.[1] This contrasts with the US, where teen births are about nineteen per thousand.[2] Key differences between European and American approaches to sexuality education involve the breadth and scope of the information taught in schools, as well as the openness and honesty of parental conversations about sexuality. For example, many US students receive education on "how to say no" to sex, but often receive little to no education about birth control.

In Europe, effective comprehensive sexuality education also typically starts young. Starting as early as in kindergarten, sex ed has proven effective at producing positive health-related outcomes. For example, in the Netherlands comprehensive sexuality education is mandated in primary schools and the government reports that most teens experience positive first sexual experiences (as opposed to most Americans reporting negative ones), and the majority of teens use contraception during their first sexual encounter.[3] Additionally, the Netherlands reports some of the lowest rates of teen pregnancy, human immunodeficiency virus (HIV), and other sexually transmitted infections (STIs) in the world.

Nearly all approaches in the US view sexuality education as a means of "risk avoidance," but rarely if ever focus on foundational aspects for the development of healthy, mutually satisfying physical relationships (which most people will eventually hope to have). School-based curricula often consist of fear-based messaging, only including heteronormative content, and are geared only toward students who are not yet sexually active. This can limit the application and receptivity of students receiving the content even if it is offered.

Many parents rely on schools to teach their children about topics related to sexuality, and yet many states do not actually require sex education in schools. At the time of writing, only twenty-nine states in the United States mandate sexuality education, and only sixteen require instruction on condoms or contraception when sexuality or HIV/STI education is provided. Additionally, some curricula, particularly in the US, are not science-based or medically accurate and are delivered by poorly qualified facilitators. And although optimistic parents may assume children and young adults are receiving accurate information about sexuality from their medical providers, a recent investigation indicated that only one in three patients received any information about sexuality from their pediatrician, and, for those who did, the conversation lasted approximately forty seconds.

According to the Centers for Disease Control and Prevention, nineteen topics are considered "critical" components of sexual education.[4] They include:

1. Communication and negotiation skills

2. Goal-setting and decision skills

3. Creating and sustaining health and respectful relationships

4. Influences of family, peers, media, technology, and other factors on sexual risk behavior

5. Preventive care that is necessary to maintain reproductive and sexual health

6. Influencing and supporting others to avoid or reduce sexual risk behaviors

7. Benefits of being sexually abstinent

8. Efficacy of condoms

9. Importance of using condoms consistently and correctly

10. Importance of using condoms at the same time as another form of contraception to prevent both STIs and pregnancy

11. How to obtain condoms

12. How to correctly use a condom

13. Methods of contraception other than condoms

14. How to access valid and reliable information, products, and services related to HIV, STDs, and pregnancy

15. How HIV and other STIs are transmitted

16. Health consequences of HIV, other STIs, and pregnancy

17. Importance of limiting the number of sexual partners

18. Sexual orientation

19. Gender roles, gender identity, and gender expression

In the United States, the portion of the school curriculum that covers all of these topics is notably low and varies between states. And even if there are a wide breadth of topics covered in sexuality education, many programs lack appropriately skilled facilitators. Research suggests that fear-based approaches and negative framing of sexuality can have lasting consequences.[5] A more balanced and positive approach to discussing sexuality can be beneficial in forming healthy sexual relationships in adulthood. And although it may sound a bit strange to talk about "kids" and "sexual pleasure" in the same sentence, framing sexuality positively can have lasting benefits. The United Nations Educational, Scientific, and Cultural Organization (UNESCO) recommends that topics related to pleasure also be included as an important factor related to sexuality.[6] These recommendations include:

- Curricula should "state that sexual feelings, fantasies, and desires are natural and not shameful, and occur throughout life." (for ages twelve to fifteen)

- Students should "understand that sexual stimulation involves physical and psychological aspects, and people respond in different ways, at different times." (for ages twelve to fifteen)

- Curricula should inform that "engaging in sexual behaviors should feel pleasurable and comes with associated responsibilities for one's health and well-being." (for age fifteen and up)

Sexuality education in schools often neglects content related to navigating relationships (other than just identifying healthy vs. unhealthy), complex components of consent, sexual behaviors other than vaginal intercourse, sexual pleasure or other reasons that people engage in sexual intercourse, and understanding personal sexual response. Because of the absence of these critical topics, not only does traditional sexuality education leave out large groups of individuals and their behaviors, but it also fails to support children in eventually becoming sexually healthy adults.

Many experts agree that a rights-based, comprehensive approach to sexuality education (CSE) is the most effective approach to equip youth with the knowledge, skills, attitudes, and values necessary to determine and enjoy their sexuality from a physical and emotional perspective (both individually and within relationships). This approach goes beyond just preventing pregnancy or disease.

Though some school-based educational programs provide a comparatively complete, medically accurate, age-appropriate sex education that is culturally congruent and responsive to the needs of young people (Personal Responsibility Education Program, or PREP), political influence has led to many states and school districts adopting abstinence-only-until-marriage-based curricula (also called Sexual Risk Avoidance). Although many parents likely support the idea of abstinence, these programs have largely been deemed ineffective and even harmful. A recent study examining the impact of US abstinence-only education programs found that they were not only ineffective at achieving their own stated goals, but that the impacts were particularly negative in terms of teenage pregnancy rates in conservative states.[7]

A more comprehensive approach to sexual education can have many benefits. A growing body of research indicates that, when exposed to a comprehensive sexuality education, kids experience:

- improved academic success

- lesser rates of child sexual abuse, dating violence, and bullying

- healthier relationships

- delayed sexual initiation

- reduced unintended pregnancy, HIV, and other STIs

- reduced sexual health disparities among lesbian, gay, bisexual, transgender, queer and questioning (LGBTQ+) youth[8]

Effective sexuality education can and should come from a variety of sources including school and home.

Parent-Child Sex Communication

In addition to school-based sexuality education, youth can benefit from positive and culturally congruent parent-child sexual communication. This involves thoughtful consideration and effective articulation of the culturally specific values and expectations that parents may have in addition to presenting sex as a normal, healthy part of personhood.

Data suggests that parents can have an influential role in adolescents' sexual behavior and decision-making. Parental behaviors and the nature of the parent/child relationship can have an impact on adolescent risk behaviors, including condom use, the number of sexual partners a child has if sexually active, and age of initiation of sex. Because of this potentially powerful impact, it is important for parents or trusted adults not only to talk to children about sex but also to consider the content and timing of those discussions.

Although parents may have a limited ability to change the information that their children are exposed to in school, they do have control over the conversations that occur at home. Parents who have frequent and open conversations can increase the likelihood that their children will have positive health outcomes in childhood and in adulthood. And that openness can have broader impacts. "Connectedness," or having a sense of being cared for, supported, and belonging (including with parents or caregivers) is considered a "protective factor" that can reduce the risk of youth engaging in risky sexual behaviors. Recent findings published in *Pediatrics* suggest that "youth that feel connected at school and home were found to be 66 percent less likely to experience health risk behaviors related to sexual health, substance use, violence, and mental health in adulthood." [9]

According to recent findings, several parenting processes—including parental monitoring, support, role modeling, and sexual communication—can have significant influence on adolescents' sexual attitudes, beliefs, and behaviors. Communicating effectively about sexual risk can have a significant influence on adolescents' attitudes, beliefs, and behaviors related to risk of and prevention of STIs and HIV.[10]

Even though having frequent and comprehensive conversations about sexuality can have many benefits, several factors can get in the way of effective Parent-Child Sex Communication. One commonly cited example is simply *parental resistance* to talking about sex. Socio-cultural differences (intergenerational differences in values, exposures, and ideas) between parents and children can also create a barrier to effective communication, in addition to fear from children of parental retribution. This book aims to assist parents in overcoming some of those challenges.

Many adults may remember having the awkward "the birds and the bees" talk with their parents or maybe even the equally embarrassing puberty discussion. Likely, those two conversations (if they even happened) captured the entire "home sex ed curriculum." But the "one and done" approach to sexuality education and expectations around sexuality often leave youth with many unanswered questions and feelings of shame about sexual development and feelings.

Modern Challenges

One challenge that youth face in their development is the quantity and quality of the messaging that they receive concerning sexuality. Even at an early age, children are exposed to explicit sexual content: messages about sexuality are embedded into video games, music, advertising, and social media. Youth also have access to pornography through the internet in a way that previous generations did not experience, and parental monitoring of exposure is difficult, if not impossible. According to recent research published in *Pediatrics* journal, 42 percent of internet users between the ages of ten and seventeen had been exposed to online pornography in the last year.[11] Of those who been exposed, 66 percent reported "only unwanted exposure" (referring mostly to shared unsolicited pictures and emails or shared files).

Although it is difficult to identify the cause-and-effect relationship between exposure to pornography in youth and its impact, we can expect that young people may get ideas about what bodies "should" look like, what sex "should" be, and what they "should" expect from sex. As young minds are developing and learning to process information critically, it would be reasonable to assume that they may not be able to process those messages in the same way that adults do.

Another challenge that youth and parents alike face is the changing landscape around issues of consent. The #MeToo movement was originally created by Tarana Burke in 2006 and eventually reached its media peak in 2017 with the sexual abuse allegations against Harvey Weinstein; it unearthed a desperate need to do a better job of educating people about sexual consent—not only to avoid legal ramifications, but to also prepare young people to interact with peers in a healthy and respectful manner. This movement has also contributed to a variety of law and policy changes that impact youth and adults, which parents may not feel equipped to discuss.

Parents may also feel ill-equipped to discuss sex with youth who are already sexually active. Sexuality education in schools is largely focused on preventing sexual behavior in students who have not already had sex. Data suggests this may be an unreasonable assumption and a shortsighted approach. According to the Guttmacher Institute, "about one in five fifteen-year-olds and two-thirds of eighteen-year-olds reported having had sex."[12] Additionally, 45 percent of adolescents aged fifteen to nineteen reported having had oral sex with a different-sex partner, and 9 percent reported having had anal sex (the riskiest type of sex contact in terms of disease transmission). It is realistic to be armed with the tools to have discussions with young people who are not sexually active as well as those who may be engaging in sexual activity.

Goal and Structure of the Book

This book aims to educate parents and guardians about key issues involving sexual health so that they may be better equipped to engage in comprehensive, age-appropriate, evidence-based, informed discussions with their children in order to optimize sexual health and reduce risk behaviors across their childhood development into young adulthood.

Readers will be exposed to various topics related to sexual health through a scientific, evidence-based, medically accurate lens. Parents can then engage in conversations armed with accurate information and more confidence.

The book also aims to take a more inclusive approach to sexuality, capturing the diverse and unique concerns and questions related to modern sexuality, including issues related to social media and the internet, topics related to consent and personal safety, unique concerns in the LGBTQ+ community, safety optimization for those who choose to be sexually active, effective abstinence promotion, and access to appropriate healthcare resources and information.

Each chapter, written in an accessible format and aimed at educating parents with little to no background in sexuality-related topics, will offer relevant information that may include the following: scientific content basics for adults, facts versus myths, and what kids need to know. At the end of the book, an age-appropriate checklist of discussion suggestions will help parents know which topics are appropriate to talk about with kids and when.

This book will give parents the tools to develop open and honest communication with their children about sexuality, free from shame, pseudoscience, and fear tactics. This book is appropriate for all types of families, and parents with children of all ages.

CHAPTER ONE

·······························

Sexuality

Keeping It Real about the "Private Parts"

One of my favorite episodes of my favorite television show (*I'm Sorry*, created by and starring Andrea Savage) follows the lead character's struggle to decide whether she should fire her very competent babysitter after hearing her refer to female sexual anatomy as "front tushy." She hilariously goes on to describe how much confusion could result if kids all grew up learning about their sexual anatomy that way. Although this show is a fictional comedy, the theme explored is one that is legitimate.

Many parents choose to use euphemisms or childish names (read: "pee pee," "wee wee," "jajay," "special parts," etc.) to describe sexual anatomy and sexual acts, in an attempt to make talking about sex with young people less intimidating. And certainly, there is no shortage of slang terms to describe sex and anatomy (as I write this, I am reading an article in *Cosmopolitan* magazine called "Here are 101 different names for boobs"). Additionally, many adults are quite uneducated about proper terminology when it comes to sexuality. However, there are many benefits to both understanding sexual anatomy and physiology and using the proper terminology to describe them.

Although some consider frank conversations with the very young about sexuality to be inappropriate, many medical professionals and sex-abuse prevention educators encourage parents to speak plainly to children about anatomy, including accurate terminology concerning sexual anatomy.[13] This can be an important component of teaching personal safety and autonomy and can also help when addressing issues surrounding consent. Many educators believe that speaking plainly, or using "standard dialect" for body parts, can empower youth in a variety of ways, including their being more comfortable talking about sexuality, discussing issues of sexual abuse, and asking adults questions.[14] Some evidence suggests that it can also promote positive body image, self-confidence, and better parent-child communication. Children who are well versed in sexual anatomy are also more skilled at navigating conversations with medical professionals and can more comfortably explain medical issues. Plain language also helps to dissuade feelings of shame associated with sexual development.

Though discussions about anatomy might be a little uncomfortable at first, young people are often very interested in what is "normal." The reality is that everyone's sexual anatomy is a bit different. When your child was born, the doctor probably assigned them a "sex" based on their sexual anatomy. Children whose assigned sex and gender identity are the same are considered cisgender. When an individual feels that their assigned sex and gender identity are different, they will sometimes refer to themselves as transgender or trans. There are also individuals who have sexual anatomy that doesn't fall into the typical categories of male or female, who are sometimes described or referred to as intersex. Each of these terms will be discussed further in Chapter Three. *Note that the descriptions provided below use the limited terms "female" and "male," which only refer to sex assigned at birth. Some individuals with a penis may not describe themselves as male and some individuals with a uterus may not describe themselves as female.*

Female Sexual Anatomy

Vulva

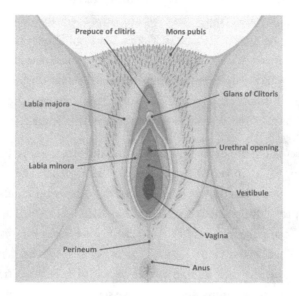

When describing female sexual anatomy, many people refer to all parts collectively as "the vagina." However, the area that most refer to as the vagina isn't that at all. The external female sex organs are known collectively as the vulva. The vulva is made up of the labia, clitoris, introitus, and the opening of the urethra.

Mons Pubis

The external, fatty area below the abdomen in the front of the vulva where many females grow most of their pubic hair after puberty is called the mons. It covers and protects the public bone. It also protects a woman's sexual organs, urinary opening, vestibule, and vagina. In some women and girls, the mons is flat and in some it is rounder. Both are normal variations. The lower part of the mons divides into a cleft that separates the mons and the labia majora.

Labia Majora

The cleft extends to form the external "lips" of the vulva called the labia majora. The labia majora also can be a variety of sizes and can swell and change color during sexual arousal. They are usually fleshy and covered with pubic hair after reaching puberty unless it is removed.

Labia Minora

Inside of the labia majora are the labia minora, or inner lips. There is great variation in what "normal" looks like. They are often referred to as the smaller lips, but can vary greatly in size, shape, and color. Sometimes the labia minora can protrude outside of the labia majora, which is also a normal variation. The labia minora can also vary in size and from each other. They can be pink, red, brown, or even purple in color. They originate at the clitoris and end at the introitus (opening of the vagina) and swell and become engorged with sexual arousal.

Glans of the Clitoris and Prepuce of the Clitoris

The labia minora connect to form foreskin, or a clitoral hood. This is tissue that covers what is typically the most sexually sensitive part of a woman's body—the clitoris. The clitoris is composed of two vestibular bulbs, the clitoral shaft, and the glans (the tip that is usually visible). It is made of spongy tissue that becomes swollen with sexual arousal. Many mistakenly believe that the visible portion of the clitoris, the glans, is the entire organ. But in reality, the clitoris is significantly larger than is externally visible. It is sensitive to stimulation during partnered sexual contact and during masturbation, with more sensory nerve endings than the penis or any other part of the human body.

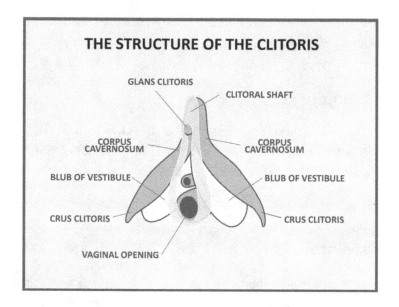

THE STRUCTURE OF THE CLITORIS

GLANS CLITORIS

CLITORAL SHAFT

CORPUS CAVERNOSUM

CORPUS CAVERNOSUM

BLUB OF VESTIBULE

BLUB OF VESTIBULE

CRUS CLITORIS

CRUS CLITORIS

VAGINAL OPENING

Urethral Opening

Just below the clitoris is the urethral opening. This is a small opening from which urine leaves the body.

Introitus and Hymen

Below the urethra is the vaginal opening, or the introitus. The vaginal opening may or may not contain additional tissue called the hymen. If present, the hymen can vary considerably in its presentation and may change over time and with activity. Though people refer to the hymen when they talk about "popping someone's cherry," it is a misleading and possibly fear-inducing analogy, as it tends to wear over time and doesn't suddenly disappear. The hymen was historically used as an "assurance" of virginity; however, due to menstruation, tampon use, physical activity, and anatomical differences, it is impossible to assess virginity through assessment of presence of hymen tissue. Though some still believe erroneously that the presence of a hymen is a "marker of virginity" and even examine it in medical and private settings, it simply isn't. According to a recent statement by the WHO, UN Human Rights Council, and UN Women, "virginity testing" has no scientific or clinical basis as there is no examination that can prove that a girl or woman has had sex, and these organizations classify the practice as a violation of the human rights of girls and women—one that can be "detrimental to women's and girls' physical, psychological and social well-being."[15]

If the hymen is present, it can vary greatly in forms. Some of those types of hymen are described and pictured below:

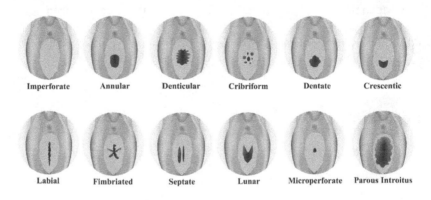

| Imperforate | Annular | Denticular | Cribriform | Dentate | Crescentic |

| Labial | Fimbriated | Septate | Lunar | Microperforate | Parous Introitus |

Microperforate hymen: a thin membrane that almost completely covers the introitus. This type of hymen may allow menstrual blood to pass but will often make tampon insertion, pelvic exams, and sexual activity difficult. A minor surgery may be required to allow for free flow of menstrual blood and to allow for tampon use.

Imperforate hymen: a thin membrane that completely covers the introitus and does not allow menstrual blood to pass through the vaginal canal and can make tampon use, pelvic exams, and sexual activity difficult. Individuals with this condition may experience back and abdominal and back pain. Treatment involves minor surgery to allow blood to pass and create an appropriately sized vaginal opening.

Septate hymen: a thin band of extra tissue that creates two openings in the introitus. The presence of a septate hymen may require minor surgery to remove the tissue, allow for insertion and removal of tampons, and create a more desirably sized vaginal opening.

Cribriform hymen: a thin membrane with many small holes in it that covers the introitus. The holes typically allow menstrual blood to pass, but can make tampon use, pelvic exams, and sexual activity difficult.

Annular hymen: a ring-shaped membrane surrounding the vaginal opening (introitus). Masturbation, tampon use, physical exertion, or sexual activity may widen the opening and reduce the presence of this type of hymen.

Parous introitus: the opening to the vagina present in a woman who has given birth to one or more children.

Perineum

In females, the perineum is the small flesh between the vagina and the anus.

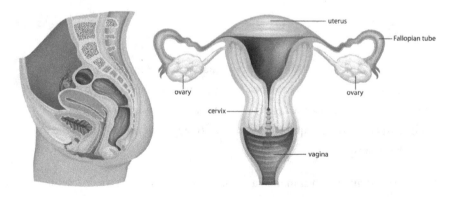

Vagina

The vagina is the internal part of the female sexual anatomy that lies beyond the introitus. It is a muscular tube that leads to the cervix, uterus, and fallopian tubes. The most sexually sensitive part of the vaginal canal exists on the lower third (the part closest to the outside of the body). When unaroused, the walls of the vagina remain pretty much "closed." With insertion (and arousal), the walls expand to accommodate a variety of sizes of objects, both in length and width.

Cervix

The cervix is the lower part of the uterus and separates it from the vaginal canal. During intercourse, sperm must pass through the opening in the cervix to fertilize an egg. Several methods of contraception, like cervical caps, female condoms, and cervical diaphragms, cover the cervix in order to prevent the passage of sperm.

Infection of the cervix by the human papillomavirus (HPV) can cause cellular changes that can progress to cervical cancer. The cervix changes in position, texture, and size under the influence of estrogen.

Uterus

The uterus is a muscular organ in females that resides in the pelvic cavity and contains the developing fetus in childbearing women. It is a pear-shaped organ in which the broad part of the "pear" is the corpus and the narrow part is the cervix.

Fallopian Tubes

The fallopian tubes are thin rods that extend laterally from the uterus toward the ovaries, which allows passage of the egg from the ovaries toward the uterus, and sperm in the opposite direction. There is one fallopian tube on either side of the uterus.

Fimbriae

The fimbriae are fingerlike projections that extend from the opening of the fallopian tubes through which eggs move from the ovary to the uterus.

Ovaries

Ovaries are the organs in females in which eggs are produced and ripened. In most girls and women, each ovary is responsible for about the same number of ovulation cycles. The ovaries also secrete hormones including estrogen, testosterone, and progesterone which help to regulate the menstrual cycle and fertility. In the ovaries, females are born with all of the oocytes (immature eggs) that they will ever have.

Bartholin's Glands

The Bartholin's glands are two small, pea-shaped glands that secrete mucus to lubricate the vagina during sexual arousal.

Skene's Glands

The Skene's glands are located near the lower end of the urethra in women and secrete fluid during sexual arousal. The Skene's glands have many similar attributes to the male prostate gland.

Breast Anatomy

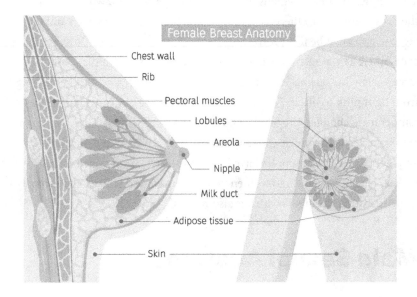

Breasts rest above the ribs and chest muscles and are made up of fifteen to twenty sections called lobes. Each lobe has lobules that end in dozens of tiny bulbs that can produce milk (in females, or people who have uteruses). The lobes, lobules, and bulbs are linked by ducts. The ducts lead to the center of the breast in the structure called the areola. Between the lobules and ducts are clusters of fat. Breast also contain blood vessels—lymph vessels that lead to lymph nodes under the arm, above the collarbone, and in the chest.

Breast changes occur throughout the lifecycle. The rate of breast growth varies greatly between young women, and the resulting breast size is also varied. Some women will experience stretch marks on the breasts during puberty, pregnancy, breastfeeding, or with weight gain. Breasts also vary in size within individuals as well. Swelling, pain, and tenderness just prior to menstruation, as well as breast texture changes during menstruation, are common as well.

Nipples and Areola

The nipples are raised regions of tissue on the breast from which milk leaves the breast through lactiferous ducts in women who have children and breast feed. Nipples can be flat, protruding, inverted, or can even be different from each other. The areola is the pigmented area around the nipple. There is a large variety in "normal" in terms of color of the nipple and areola, ranging from light pink to black. The areola and nipple color can also change due to temperature changes, pregnancy and lactation, and with age. The size of the areola varies just as much and may also change in size with breast growth and lactation. Mature nipples have lactiferous ducts from which milk is released during lactation in women. Some women also will also have hair growth around the areola which is also normal.

Male Sexual Anatomy

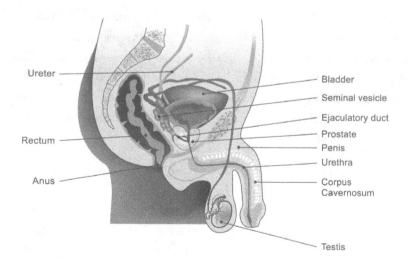

Shaft of the Penis

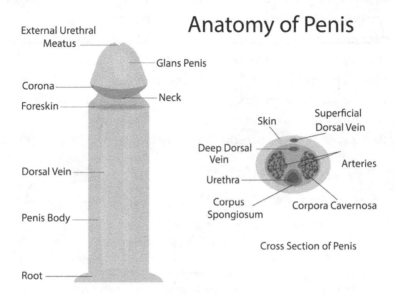

Anatomy of Penis

External Urethral Meatus

Glans Penis

Corona

Neck

Foreskin

Dorsal Vein

Penis Body

Root

Skin

Superficial Dorsal Vein

Deep Dorsal Vein

Arteries

Urethra

Corpus Spongiosum

Corpora Cavernosa

Cross Section of Penis

The penis is the organ that allows for genital intercourse and provides a channel for urine to leave the body. It gets its cylindrical shape due to its composition of three layers of spongy tissue (the corpus cavernosa and corpus spongiosum) that swell during sexual arousal. With sexual stimulation, the muscles around the arteries relax and allow more blood to fill into the penis, causing the tissue to become engorged and creating an erection (or a "hard-on" or "boner"). Despite the name, there is no bone in the penis that creates an erection. Penises vary greatly in size, with the average erect penis measuring five to seven inches. There can be great change in the size of a flaccid penis when it becomes erect, or not much change at all. Some penises are very straight while erect, while others have a slight or pronounced curvature. Some curvature is due to normal variation but can also be caused by trauma or other medical conditions.

Glans

The glans of the penis is the sensitive tip. It is filled with nerve endings that are particularly sensitive to sexual stimulation. Two of the most sensitive parts of the glans are the frenulum (a thin band of skin on its underside connecting the glans with the shaft, that looks like a small v just below the head of the penis) and the corona (the ridge around the edge of the glans). At birth, the glans of the penis is covered by tight foreskin which usually loosens with maturation. In uncircumcised males, the glans is covered by foreskin in its flaccid state. With erection, the foreskin retracts, and the glans is exposed.

To circumcise or not to circumcise?

Male circumcision is the surgical removal of the skin that covers the glans of the penis. This procedure is fairly common and varies in popularity by country, tradition, and religious practice. The procedure is most commonly performed during infancy but can be performed later in life. The American Academy of Pediatrics leaves the decision to circumcise up to the parents, though they highlight several benefits. Circumcision may have various health benefits, including:[16]

- Enhanced Hygiene

- Decreased risk of urinary tract infections

- Decreased risk of contracting and passing sexually transmitted infections

- Decreased risk of penile cancer

- Decreased risk of penile problems like phimosis (difficult or impossible to retract foreskin)

Urinary Meatus

The urinary meatus is the opening at the tip of the glans that allows for urine, pre-ejaculate, and semen to exit the body. It presents as a vertical slit.

Scrotum

The scrotum is a pouch-like sac of skin that contains the testicles and many nerves and blood vessels. The scrotum can vary in size, hairiness, and color. They are typically very sensitive. The scrotum helps to maintain proper temperature of the testicles where sperm is produced. Muscles in the wall of the scrotum contract or relax to move the testicles closer to the body for warmth or further away from the body to cool.

Testicles

The testicles (testes) are male gonads that reside in the scrotum. Most men have two of these organs that produce testosterone and sperm. Testicles vary in size. The testes are filled with coiled seminiferous tubules where sperm cells are produced.

Epididymis and Vas Deferens

The epididymis is a coiled tube that serves to help bring sperm to maturity and assists with carriage and storage of sperm cells that are produced in the testes. During sexual arousal, contractions force the sperm from the epididymis to the ejaculatory ducts through the vas deferens (partially coiled muscular tube which exits the abdominal cavity through the inguinal canal).

Urethra

The urethra is a tube that carries urine from the bladder and semen (in males) to the outside of the body. During erection, urine flow is blocked, allowing only semen to be released during orgasm.

Prostate Gland

The prostate gland functions to provide fluid to ejaculate and provide liquid that helps to nourish sperm. It is a walnut-shaped gland that surrounds part of the urethra. It changes in size throughout the lifecycle.

Seminal Vesicles

The seminal vesicles attach to the vas deferens near the base of the bladder and add fluids to ejaculate. They produce a sugar-rich liquid that aids in sperm mobility. Fluid produced by the seminal vesicles makes the majority of the volume of male ejaculate.

Bulbourethral Glands

Bulbourethral glands, also called Cowper's glands, produce fluid that lubricates the urethra and helps to neutralize any acidity that may be present in the urethra due to the passage of urine.

Intersex Sexual Anatomy

Intersex is sometimes used as a general term to describe individuals born with reproductive anatomy that doesn't fit the "typical" definitions of male or female. There is great variation in what "counts" as intersex which makes it difficult to state its prevalence in general terms. These individuals may have genitals that seem "in between" like an unusually large clitoris, the lack of a vaginal opening, an unusually small penis, or a scrotum that is divided so that it resembles labia. They may have mostly male-typical anatomy on the inside and female-typical anatomy on the outside or vice versa. The person may have some cells with XX chromosome and some having XY.

CHAPTER TWO

....

Puberty
"What in the World Is Going On Here?"

Puberty

The day I started my first period, I was at a church youth-group retreat, staying at a small cabin in the middle of nowhere. I had just turned thirteen and do not remember having ever discussed "periods" (cue teenage shudder) with any adult. After noticing that something didn't feel right, I excused myself to the rustic bathroom, and, upon discovery, went into an instant panic. I still had several days left on the retreat and had (obviously) not come prepared. I frantically started rifling in the under-sink cabinet (that belonged to some elderly woman from our church who had been kind enough to donate the use of her cabin, and whom I am sure hadn't menstruated since the early seventies). When I finally found a pad, it was so old-fashioned that it was designed to be used with a belt. I eventually helped myself to this poor woman's stash and used some sort of MacGyver methodology to make do with this foreign, pad-like contraption. My tiny, eighty-ish-pound frame was not designed to hide this humungous old-fashioned relic, what to me felt like a small mattress in my underwear. And, keeping true to form with church retreats, the rest of the weekend was packed with "team building" games that involved every possible awkward position that made hiding this massive annoyance nearly impossible. This was long before the days of cell phones, and I didn't dare disclose my secret to anyone at the retreat. Certainly "Christians" didn't talk about menstruation! I remember thinking, *THIS is what women have to put up with?!* For months, I was full of great dread, missing my carefree, pre-period days.

Likely every adult remembers with great clarity their "puberty story." It can be a fairly traumatic process for some, particularly if unprepared. (I am often reminded of Brooke Shields in *The Blue Lagoon* when I talk about puberty, and I think about how scary it must be to have a period for the first time having no knowledge of what is going on.) Understanding what to expect as children go through puberty can help parents cope with the mental and emotional changes that occur and can help reduce the anxiety for young people as they anticipate and grapple with the changes.

Girls (or Those Born with a Uterus)

Puberty is a time of great sexual and physical maturation. The age that young people start the process of puberty can vary greatly and can be the cause of great concern among adolescents. Trends indicate that puberty is beginning at younger ages in girls when compared to previous generations. There are likely a variety of factors that contribute to this trend, including childhood obesity and environmental circumstances. Preparing kids for what to expect can make the stressful process more comfortable and can ease some of their concerns.

In general, girls start puberty at ages eight to thirteen, earlier than boys by about a couple years. Puberty in girls is usually described by many as starting with menstruation, but it is actually marked by a cumulative set of changes that happen in gradual stages. It signifies the development of secondary sex characteristics, sexual maturation, and (in many) reproductive ability. When a girl starts puberty later, it may be that she is just a "late bloomer" or could indicate glandular or other conditions. If there are concerns, it may be appropriate to contact a medical provider. Early (precocious) puberty can be signified by very rapid body changes before the eighth birthday, and these body changes often appear out of order (i.e., menstruation before breast development). If those signs occur, it is advisable to speak to a medical professional.

Researchers and medical professionals use the "Tanner Scale" to describe stages of physical development including of the breasts, genitals, testicular volume, and public hair.[17] According to a recent population-based study on puberty published in *Paediatric and Perinatal Epidemiology*, the data indicated that girls, on average, got their first period at age 13.0 and reached Tanner Breast Stage 5 at 15.8 years (breast reaches final adult size; areola returns to contour of the surrounding breast, with a projecting central papilla[18]). Daughters in the study had menarche (first period) an average of 3.6 months earlier than their mothers had.

Some changes that girls can expect to accompany puberty are described below. It is important to note that these changes are individual and happen at different times for each girl. Girls may also advance through the stages differently.

Physiological changes in girls (those born with a uterus) during puberty:

- Development of breast buds: Small mounds form under the nipple, and the breast and nipple become slightly raised. The areola will increase in size.

- Breast growth: The breast will increase in size and become more rounded and fuller.

- Nipple and areola development: The nipple and areola will again become raised, forming another mound.

- Public hair growth: Public hair growth will often start as long, soft hair in a small space around the genitals.

- Expanded pubic hair growth: Pubic hair is darker and course. It resembles adult hair and spreads, even to the thighs and stomach.

Additional changes may include:

- Increase in hair growth: Young women will often experience an increase in hair in the underarm area and on the legs. Some feel comfortable removing this hair and some choose to leave it.

- Body shape changes: Puberty often facilitates fairly dramatic changes in bodily appearance. For many, there will be an increase in height and weight, and body shape may change, especially in the hips, legs, buttocks, and stomach.

- Seemingly disproportionate growth spurts: During puberty, some may find that feet, arms, legs, and hands grow disproportionately with the rest of the body. This may add to feelings of awkwardness and make young people feel clumsy for a period of time.

- Skin changes: Hormonal changes that accompany puberty can create bothersome changes to the skin, particularly that of the face, chest, upper back, and shoulders. Acne is fairly common. Increased sweating and oily skin may occur. Daily face washing and showering are important to address these issues.

- Labia changes: During puberty, the labia may change in color and grow larger.

- Menstruation: Most girls will begin having menstrual periods and begin ovulation in the early teen years. This occurs when the ovaries begin ripening eggs and the lining of the uterus develops in order to prepare for reproduction. If the egg ripened and released during ovulation is not fertilized, menstruation (or the shedding of the lining of the uterus) will occur. If the egg is fertilized, pregnancy will occur. Menstrual periods are typically sporadic in the early stages and become more regular over time. Periodic vaginal discharge, both clear and slightly whitish, is a normal part of the maturation process.

Boys (or Those Born with a Penis)

Just like in girls, puberty happens in a boy in series of stages. One part of that series is the development of secondary sex characteristics. Boys typically start puberty later than girls, typically ranging from ages nine to fourteen. It is important to note that age of puberty onset varies. According to a recent population-based study on puberty, published in *Paediatric and Perinatal Epidemiology*, voice-breaking in boys occurs at an average age of 13.1, first ejaculation of semen at 13.4, and Tanner Genital Stage 5 at 15.6 (testicular volume greater than 20 ml; adult scrotum and penis, pictured as last stage below on the far right).[19]

Additional physical changes that occur in boys during puberty are described below.

Physiological changes in boys during puberty:

- Enlargement of the scrotum and testes: The earliest change that characterizes puberty in boys is the growth of the scrotum and testes without significant growth of the penis. Following that period of growth, the penis will begin to grow along with continued growth of the scrotum and testes.

- Early pubic hair growth: The first signs of pubic hair will appear in a small area around the genitals and will be relatively sparse, long, soft hair.

- Changing of pubic hair: With maturation, public hair will become darker and coarser. It will continue to spread and cover a larger area of the body and may spread up the stomach and to the thighs.

Additional changes may include:

- Seemingly disproportionate growth spurts: The feet, arms, legs, and hands may seem to "outgrow" the rest of the body for a time. They may cause feelings of clumsiness and awkwardness.

- Swelling in the breast area: Hormonal changes during puberty may cause temporary swelling. This is typically a short-term condition. Seek medical guidance if there is concern.

- Voice changes: Cracking and deepening of the voice typically occurs during puberty. The cracking is typically temporary.

- Hair growth: Boys will often develop hair growth in the underarm area, legs, and face, as well as continued hair growth around the genital area.

- Skin changes: Oily skin, increased sweating, and stronger odor in sweat typically occurs as a result of hormonal changes that accompany puberty. Face washing, deodorant use, and daily showering are particularly important.

- Erections: Frequent erections due to hormonal changes are common during puberty. They can occur as a result of sexual fantasies, physical stimulation, or can happen involuntarily. They commonly happen upon first waking and can occur in the night and be accompanied by ejaculation (wet dreams).

- Sperm production: Sperm production begins during puberty and marks the capacity for reproduction. Semen is expelled during ejaculation and is made up of sperm and other fluids.

Emotional Changes of Puberty

- Mood swings: Increased hormone levels during puberty often cause fluctuations in mood and feelings of intense emotion. Mood changes may feel random and have rapid onset.

- Sexual thoughts and urges: Feelings of romantic and sexual attraction are common during puberty. It is normal to feel attracted to males, females, or both. Masturbation is normal and common and may even help people to explore their sexuality to determine what they do and do not like.

- Body image and appearance concerns: It is normal to start feeling more preoccupied with personal appearance in adolescence. Preoccupation with being a "late bloomer" or "early bloomer" can add to stress of this life stage.

- Craving privacy: It is normal for teens to begin to yearn for more privacy and independence from their parents as they begin to establish themselves as individuals.

- Worry about the future: Brain development that occurs in the teenage years allows young people to start thinking about their futures and more abstract concepts. Some may start to worry about things like school violence, politics, divorce of parents, friendships, etc.

- Self-conscious feelings: Teens' emotions often appear exaggerated. Sulking and outbursts are common. Being embarrassed to be seen with parents and pulling away from things associated with childhood are common. Kids in this stage may resist being hugged or kissed by their parents or other family members.

- Expression experimentation: Teens are changing rapidly and often will begin to experiment with new ways of expressing themselves. This may include new interests, new ways of talking or acting, and "trying on" different strategies of moving through life.

- Experimentation with long-term commitments: as teenagers begin to struggle with independence, they often will describe being "in love" and committing to long-term relationships.

Cognitive Changes of Puberty

- Changes in reasoning and thinking: Children in this stage begin to make notable maturational leaps in the way they think, reason, and learn. Children are starting to comprehend more abstract ideas and are able to think about things and ideas they can't see. They are more able to problem-solve and see consequences. They are more capable at considering multiple perspectives.

- Changes in thinking: Young teens are better able to learn advanced and complex topics. Their ability for more complex learning and reasoning allows them to anticipate how others might react to them and things that they do. They may attempt more manipulation of parents as they are better capable of anticipating consequences of actions.

- Identity formation: Teens will go through "phases" of exploration, experimenting with a variety of identities. This is a normal and even healthy part of adolescence. They also become more aware of their roles as student, son or daughter, friend, etc.

- Dichotomous actions and thoughts: Teens may display a variety of behaviors that appear at odds with their goals and ideals. Although they may feel strongly and passionately about something, they also lack the maturity and experience to "act like adults."

Ways Parents Can Provide Support to Kids as They Go through Puberty

- Reassure: Emphasize that the changes are normal and happen in their own time. Some changes (like the slight growth of breast tissue that some boys experience) can create great anxiety for young people. Talk to them about fact-based changes that occur and consider leaving them evidence-based reading materials to explore on their own. Focus on the positive aspects of maturation and transition to adulthood.

- Show compassion: Many of the mood swings and what feels like irrational emotional responses are temporary. Be patient and understanding. This too shall pass.

- Prepare: Prior to having their first period, talk to your child about menstrual products and purchase supplies that they can take with them to school and keep in their bathroom at home, and, if they stay at places other than your home (with another parent or guardian), consider getting supplies to leave there as well.

- Offer praise: Make a point of reinforcing positive behaviors and accomplishments.

- Seek support: Develop a circle of friends who can act as a support system. Connecting with other parents of teenagers can reinforce the "normalcy" of this time and provide an outlet for parents during what can be a frustrating time for all concerned.

- Encourage good hygiene: Emphasizing the importance of daily showers, face washing, and deodorant use is important. This will help your children to stay healthy, as well as improve their social connections.

- Support self-expression: Trying on new identities is a healthy part of puberty. Encourage kids to try different things and resist the urge to discourage them as they "try on" new identities, including hair styles and clothing choices that may seem odd to you.

- Respect privacy: Try to be tolerant of teens' desire for privacy, including long hours of seclusion in their bedroom and bathroom. Set limits that are reasonable for the family.

- Seek professional care if concerned: If you are concerned with your child's acne, seek out a skin specialist or dermatologist. If you are concerned that their sullen behavior or mood swings are beyond the normal changes that occur in the teen years, it may be advised to reach out to a mental health care professional.

CHAPTER THREE

Sexual Orientation and Gender Identity

Respecting and Understanding Differences

Some people may find it difficult to talk about gender identity and sexual orientation because they feel limited by a lack of understanding or familiarity with the language surrounding those topics. An important part of creating a sex-positive home is fostering respect and understanding of all people. Prejudice and discrimination against people who identify as gay, lesbian, or bisexual can have serious mental health consequences. Developing a greater understanding of sexual orientation and identities as well as improving vocabulary within those topics can help to foster respect of all persons and can help us to communicate more effectively and respectfully.

Sexual Orientation

Sexual Orientation is defined as an inherent or immutable enduring emotional, romantic, or sexual attraction to other people, including men, women, or both. Sexual orientation is defined in relation to others and defines the group of people in which one is likely to find satisfying and fulfilling romantic relationships. It is often described erroneously by many as an "either, or" state of being (i.e., homosexual or heterosexual, gay or straight), but that is inappropriately discrete and polarized. Some may describe themselves as *heterosexual* (physically, spiritually, emotionally attracted to those of a different sex), *homosexual* (physically, spiritually, emotionally attracted to those of the same sex), *bisexual* (physically, spiritually, emotionally attracted to those of the same sex and a different sex) or *asexual* (though there are various definitions, in general, it means the person feels no sexual attraction or the intrinsic desire to have sex). Many people find it comforting to view our sexual attractions in reductionist terms, but in many ways that is problematic. A large body of research, dating back more than eighty years, supports the notion that sexual orientation is far more complex.[20]

To demonstrate this complexity, I always start my college lectures about sexual orientation with the following exercise. I start the activity by asking students to raise their hand (if they choose to participate) if they think that "someone is gay or lesbian" in each of the following scenarios. (Stick with me, it will make sense in a moment.)

- A person engages in same-sex behavior but doesn't consider themselves gay or have "romantic" relationships with people of the same sex.

- A person is a sex worker and engages in same-sex behavior for money, but only has romantic relationships with people of the opposite sex.

- A person feels romantically and sexually attracted to people of the same sex throughout their entire life and fantasizes about it, but never acts on it.

- A person finds it arousing to see members of the same sex naked in pictures, pornography, and in person, but does not consider themselves gay or engage in same-sex behavior.

As the students hear the scenarios, I always see inquisitive looks as they begin to see that traditional notions about "gay or straight" may be inappropriately limited. Three important distinctions in the scenarios described above are that they contrast in sexual *attraction*, sexual *behavior*, and sexual *orientation identity*. Some students are of the belief that possessing same-sex attraction, regardless of acting on it, makes a person "gay or lesbian." Others will state that as long as no same-sex sexual behavior has occurred, the person isn't "gay or lesbian" even if they feel romantic attraction. Still others see that limiting identities to terms like "gay or straight" is unnecessary and simply invites misunderstanding.

Sexual attraction—refers to the emotional and sexual response people feel toward another.

Sexual behavior—refers to activity (either solitary, in pairs, or with more than two people) that induces sexual arousal.

Sexual orientation identity—refers to an individual's inner awareness of themselves in terms of whom one is romantically or sexually attracted to as well as membership in a community of others who share those attractions. This may also include the choice to identify or dis-identify with a sexual orientation.

Research over many decades indicates that sexual orientation occurs along a continuum and not as an "either, or" state of being. There isn't a scientific consensus describing the reasons people develop heterosexual, bisexual, gay, lesbian, or other sexual orientations. Some believe there is a complex interaction or nature and nurture influences that shape orientation, and most people will state that they feel little or no sense of choice about their sexual orientation.

It's likely that sexual orientation involves a range of variables. One model, created by Alfred Kinsey in the 1940s, describes orientation with a "Heterosexual-Homosexual Rating Scale."[21] Kinsey described orientation in terms of experience, ranging from "exclusively heterosexual" to "predominantly heterosexual, only incidentally homosexual" to "predominantly heterosexual, but more than incidentally heterosexual" to "equally heterosexual and homosexual" to "predominantly homosexual, but more than incidentally heterosexual" to "exclusively homosexual." Later research would challenge this tool, pointing out its limitations (the scale implies that the more same-gender-oriented one is, the less heterosexual one is, and it doesn't include discussions of attraction and identification—

only behavior). Regardless of its limitations, it does highlight the nonbinary nature of sexual orientation.

According to the National Survey of Family Growth, among adolescents ages eighteen and nineteen just under 8 percent of females and just under 3 percent of males identify as homosexual or bisexual.[22] Many young people who identify as LGBTQ+ are happy and thrive. However, these adolescents are at increased risk for bullying, suicide attempts, homelessness, alcohol use, and risky sex. Parental support can be very influential in easing this process and reducing likelihood of negative mental and physical health consequences. To date, there has been no credible scientific evidence showing that therapy aimed at changing sexual orientation ("conversion therapy") is safe or effective.

How Do People Know and Form Their Sexual Orientation?

Sexual orientation is typically defined between middle childhood and early adolescence. Orientation is independent of sexual behavior, and one need not experience sexual activity in order to feel that they are lesbian, gay, bisexual, or heterosexual (or some other variation). Some people, regardless of type, will feel their sexual orientation long before acting on it, called *unexplored commitment*.[23] Some will experiment with same-sex and other-sex sexual activity (even if it differs from their identity) before "assigning a label," or may even choose to reject a label. Fear of prejudice, rejection, or discrimination can make it more difficult for people to come to terms with their sexual orientation.

The process of sexual-identity formation has been studied by researchers. According to research by Worthington et. al., *heterosexual identity* appears to happen over time and encompass six important dimensions:[24]

- Contemplation of alternative possibilities related to sexual needs, leading to the deliberate conclusion of being "heterosexual"

- Formation of value system related to sexuality and sexual behavior

- Awareness of preferred sexual activities

- Awareness of preferred partner characteristics

- Awareness of preferences regarding sexual expression

- Recognition of one's sexual orientation and personal identification with that orientation

Although also met with some later critique, research from Australian psychologist Vivienne Cass sought to explore sexual identity as an evolving entity.[25] Cass also proposed six stages of sexual-identity formation among those who form lesbian, gay, and bisexual identities. She emphasized that there are many individual variations in how different people may progress through the stages.

Stage 1: Identity Confusion—Individuals in this stage may grapple with the question, "Am I gay/lesbian/bisexual?" They may experience a sense of incongruence between the broader social narrative and their own personal view of sexual self. They may start collecting more information related to sexual identity.

Stage 2: Identity Comparison—Individuals in this stage begin to explore the broader implications of how their sexual orientation will impact relationships. They may experience positive feelings or feelings of shame and will continue to try to "pass" as heterosexual, or they may lash out with antigay actions and internalized homophobia. They may begin to engage in same-sex behavior without defining themselves as "gay."

Stage 3: Identity Tolerance—Individuals in this stage accept themselves as members of their identity groups and begin to recognize the needs associated with that identity. They may increase their involvement with the gay community and seek supportive, like-minded social ties. Persons with strong social skills and support may be more successful at this integration. Those who struggle with the social integration and lack social support are more likely to experience stress, depression, and anxiety. Some may choose to remain secretive about their identity while others may choose to "come out" and share their identity with others.

Stage 4: Identity Acceptance—In this stage, people accept their LGBTQ+ self-image, in contrast to "tolerating" it. They may become more imbedded in the culture.

Stage 5: Identity Pride—In this stage, individuals start to move away from the "heterosexual norm" of comparison. They may become more politically involved, more confrontational, and abandon attempts to "pass" as heterosexuals in any circumstance. Anger is common in this stage. Some who have spent a lifetime "in the closet" may choose to "come out" for the first time, much to the surprise of family, friends, and coworkers. Movement to the next level is largely dependent on the reactions and level of support of those around them.

Stage 6: Synthesis—In this stage, individuals realize that sexual identity is just one aspect of what defines individuals. People begin to move away from a reductionist view of humanity toward a more inclusive view. They may begin to move away from "tribal" commitments to their community, realizing that not all heterosexuals are to be viewed negatively and not all members of their orientation community are to be viewed positively. Anger dissipates and the individual can develop a richer sense of self beyond their sexual orientation.

Parents, schools, churches, peers, and communities can play a significant role in healthy personal sexual-orientation development. Progression through the identity stages in the LGBTQ+ community may be particularly challenging among those in places or groups where their identities are more stigmatized. This may be true in rural communities and among African American and Latino males. Members of those groups may benefit particularly from parental, peer, and community support.

Gender Identity

Many people use the terms "sex" and "gender" interchangeably when they are actually describing different things. One way to begin to understand this is to look at the biological underpinnings of sex.

Genetic sex—When the sperm and egg unite, a "genetic map" acts as a blueprint to direct the body to further express characteristics of maleness, femaleness, or a mix of sexual characteristics (sometimes referred to as **intersex**).

Gonadal sex—The genetic blueprint leads to the development of gonads (either ovaries or testes) which produce hormones that dictate many body changes including secondary sex characteristics later in life.

Body sex—Genes and hormones present or lacking will influence the development of internal and external sex organs. This is influenced by anatomical structures with which the person was born as well as other social and environmental factors.

Brain sex—Although we are learning all the time about the complexities of brain sex, the brain is possibly sexually differentiated by a variety of hormonal exposures during and following the prenatal period as well as other genetic factors.

As children develop, they are influenced by a variety of factors that help to shape their self-concept and identity. Cues from influential people around them begin to shape expectations about what it means to be a "girl" or a "boy." Children also become aware of their own sexual anatomy and identify them as matching expectations of "girl" or "boy" parts. Children are also socialized by parents and communities with gendered expectations that influence personal identity (dressing boys in blue and girls in pink, not allowing boys to cry, etc.). This mix of factors all work together to create a child's core gender identity, or their earliest, prepubescent inner sense of maleness, femaleness, or ambivalence. Following puberty, gender identity is confirmed as hormonal influences begin to shape sexual fantasies and self-concept. Some may feel congruence between genetic, gonadal, body, and brain sex (*cisgender*). Other may experience an incongruence. *Transgendered* youth have developed a gender identity in opposition to their gender assigned at birth. They may be physically male but experience themselves as female, or physically female but experience themselves as male. They may also experience themselves as a blend of both or neither. Gender exists on a spectrum. People who identify as *nonbinary* do not define their gender as falling within the category of male or female. *Genderqueer/genderfluid* refer to individuals who do not identify themselves as having a specific gender at all.

Gender identity is independent of sexual orientation. Gender identity (feelings about self) does not necessarily dictate who an individual will find sexually attractive (feelings toward others).

Even if sexually orientation and gender identity are confusing to you, it is important to be respectful of all people. To model this and to foster this respect in your children:

- Learn proper terminology concerning sexual orientation and gender identity.

- Don't make assumptions about a person's gender. When in doubt, ask.

- Use preferred names and preferred gender pronouns (she/her, he/him, they/them, or ze/hir, etc.). In short, just call people what they want to be called. You wouldn't call someone Sarah if they wanted to be called Jane.

- Be a friendly ally.

CHAPTER FOUR

·····································

Consent

The "Affirmative and Enthusiastic" Standard

I still remember my first crush quite vividly. More specifically, it was my first two crushes and they happened at exactly the same time. It was 1984, the objectively memorable year that the two best movies of all time were released—*Purple Rain* (the story of a breakout musician who struggles with an abusive home life and a budding, contentious romance) and *Sixteen Candles* (a coming-of-age classic that follows a sullen "just turned sixteen-year-old" through all of the usual teenage embarrassments). That year, I, like most everyone I knew, fell in love with the male leads: Jake Ryan (Michael Earl Schoeffling) and "The Kid" (Prince).

At the time, they were my standard of masculinity and male attractiveness. I found their bold and sometimes aggressive confidence to be captivating. At that point, I had very little exposure to intimate relationships, and certainly not to the "behind the scenes" of sexual relationships. But I knew that I found this chemistry and seductive power dynamic intriguing.

Although I still find them both quite dreamy, the lens through which I view their characters has changed from my naive and once idyllic perception. As my feminist lens has developed, my conception of what it means to be "masculine" as well as what a desirable partner is have also changed. Time, wisdom, parenthood, and evolving attitudes about consent have undoubtedly changed many of our perceptions of what intimate relationships and interactions should look like. One must only follow the news to see many examples of how antiquated and often sexist views of sexual consent are no longer tolerated by many in broader society.

On its surface, consent can seem like a fairly simple concept—permission for something to happen or agreeing to do something. But when we add in sexual contact to the equation, it gets a little more complicated. As the concept of sexual consent has recently received more "press" following the #MeToo movement, deeper analysis reveals the need for more nuance in our discussions and understanding.

Although many of my feminist colleagues may scoff at this statement, sexual consent can feel confusing and at times even awkward. My guess is that most of the people reading this grew up around countless examples of movies, television shows, and music that unapologetically normalized examples of nonconsensual sexual contact. In fact, I dare you to rewatch some of your favorite eighties movies and television shows targeted toward teens and count the examples of behavior that would be considered harassment, assault, or rape by today's standards. I will admit with chagrin that some of my favorite childhood classics are fairly cringeworthy to watch today. Even though few could argue that Jake Ryan was devastatingly handsome and charming in *Sixteen Candles*, many of us have probably forgotten that he bragged and stated about his passed-out girlfriend that "[he] could violate her ten different ways if [he] wanted to." And how many have forgotten that, in the classic *Revenge of the Nerds*, the leading "nerd" lures the beautiful sorority character into a sexual situation by impersonating her boyfriend and then appears to have sex with her under those false pretenses? And can you imagine the workplace dynamic between Sam and Diane on *Cheers* playing out by today's standards of workplace harassment?

Repeated exposure to those "social scripts" and gendered sexual expectations can make it feel confusing and foreign to tackle conversations about sexual consent when so many of our own exposures seem to be contradictory. With so many mixed messages and conflicting exposures, it can feel daunting to sort out what is considered "OK" and what is considered taboo or even illegal by modern standards.

Many of us were raised on the continuously reinforced narrative that sex "negotiation" includes a push and pull scripted by gender roles in which men and boys act as the nagging aggressors and women and girls act as the reluctant receivers.

Even among adults, I frequently encounter a lack of understanding about how to even define consent, the legal implications of consent, and how to go about asking for it. This lack of understanding can create barriers to having productive discussions with children about consent-related issues.

Many of us were also raised with reiterations of the notion that "no means no" in terms of relational interactions, including sexual contact. But when applied to sexual consent, teaching children (and adults) that "no means no" is simply not enough to establish enthusiastic permission to engage in sexual behavior. Historical approaches are far too simplistic and grossly inadequate to navigate the current evolving climate that demands equity and respect. Increasingly, a movement toward "enthusiastic affirmative consent" or a more "yes means yes" approach is gaining traction in educational and policy arenas. A firm understanding of how to establish consent can not only protect children and future adults from misunderstandings or even legal consequence but can also create healthier and more equitable relationships in general.

Among its many benefits, the #MeToo movement shed light on issues surrounding our understanding and practice of consent and illuminated the need to start much younger with consent education. In the words of #MeToo founder Tarana Burke, "We need to start earlier to proactively discuss the entire spectrum of violence and help shift the culture so we are preventing another generation of children from having to say, 'me too.' We have an incredible opportunity to do that with comprehensive sexuality education. Let's not waste it."

What Is Sexual Consent?

In a general sense, most would agree that asking for permission to engage in sexual contact is a reasonable expectation. And the definition of sexual consent has never really changed, but the way we talk about it and (hopefully) teach it has.

Sexual consent is agreement to participate in a sexual activity. Sexual activity without consent is sexual assault or rape. States and countries vary in their definitions of each. According to the Rape, Abuse & Incest National Network (RAINN), every seventy-three seconds, an American is sexually assaulted.[26] And every nine minutes, the victim is a child. Although sexual assault can happen to anyone, of any age and any race and socioeconomic background, teenage girls and young women are particularly vulnerable. Females ages sixteen to nineteen are four times more likely than the general population to be victims of rape, attempted rape, or sexual assault. Additionally, individuals that identify as TGQN (transgender, genderqueer, nonconforming) can be at increased risk as well.

Sexual assault and rape can include a variety of behaviors including genital touching, oral sex, and vaginal or anal penetration (with body parts or other objects). Legal and policy definitions may also vary according to country, state, county, or even by institution.

Understanding sexual consent can prevent misinterpretations and can also help young people to recognize abuse if it happens. One easy way to conceptualize sexual consent is with Planned Parenthood's description using the acronym of FRIES, summarized here:

> F—Freely given
> R—Reversible
> I—Informed
> E—Enthusiastic
> S—Specific

Consent Is Freely Given

Consent must be given without the presence of coercion, implied pressure stemming from power imbalance, manipulation, or influence of drugs and alcohol. To give consent, an individual must be acting on their own free will. This also means there is no violence or threat of violence involved in the decision-making process. It is important to note that each state has its own definition of consent, either in established law or through court cases.

It is also important to consider and further define a person's "capacity to consent." Some of the factors to consider include: a person's age, the status of the person in terms of disability, the relationship to the individual with whom they are involved in sexual contact, the person's consciousness and intoxication status, and their status as "vulnerable" according to the law.

A person who is drunk or high cannot give sexual consent. A person who is passed out or asleep or not fully awake cannot give consent. Some physical or intellectual disabilities can impede a person's capacity to give consent.

Each state will have its own laws surrounding legal age of consent. It is important to become aware of the laws in your state. In the United States, the ages range from sixteen to eighteen. Some states also have specific laws that consider the age difference in parties when determining ability to consent. In some states, if the partners are married, the younger party can consent to their spouse even if under the legal age of consent in that state. Additionally, the severity of legal punishment can be influenced by the position of authority that the older party has over the younger party (as in parent to child, teacher to student, caretaker to client, etc.). States also have different laws regarding consent as it relates to physical and intellectual disabilities which can have a significant impact on both vulnerability to sexual violence and empowerment as it relates to sexual autonomy. It may also be prudent to become aware of these laws in your state.

Before even asking for consent, it is important to understand how power differences between the parties involved might impact the ability of one to consent freely to sexual activity. When thinking about consent among parties where there may be power differences (differences in age, financial status, educational attainment, citizenship, career positionality), it is important for the person to consider, "would this person say yes if there weren't differences in power, position, or authority?" Reiterate that saying no is always ok. When in doubt, ask. If there is a power imbalance, the person may feel like there will be negative consequences if they say no. Consent is not possible when a person feels like they don't have a choice.

When asking for consent when a power imbalance exists, it is particularly important to make sure to emphasize to the person that there are options. Clearly stated questions like, "Would you like to move this to the bedroom, or would you prefer to hang out here and play cards?" can make it easier to establish if the person is acting on free will.

Consent Is Reversible

It is important to understand that consent can be revoked at any time. Just because someone gives consent one day, doesn't mean they have given consent the next day even for the same act. Even in the heat of the moment, an individual can still change their mind. It doesn't matter if the person has been flirtatious all night, what clothes they are wearing, even if they are in bed naked. Consent can be revoked at any time. Even if sexual activity was discussed and agreed upon prior to meeting, the person is entitled to change their mind.

Any time I give this talk to students or adults, I almost always have someone challenge me by referring to instances in which someone was not convicted of rape or assault despite lack of consent. There are certainly countless cases of injustice in this area, but why would anyone want to risk it?

Consent Is Informed

Consent is only possible if a person has all of the facts. If someone is told their sex partner is using birth control pills when they are not, that is not full consent. If someone is told their sex partner will use a condom and they don't, that is not full consent. If a person is misrepresenting who they are, there cannot be full consent.

Consent Is Enthusiastic

Previously accepted social scripts surrounding sexuality include passivity and silent negotiation. Many media depictions of sexually attractive men include dominance and aggression. It is not difficult to see why these messages can create confusion. But affirmative sexual consent is more than "no means no." Affirmative sexual consent means that "yes means yes." Just because someone isn't saying no, it doesn't mean that they are saying yes. Some states and college campuses even have legislation and policies requiring affirmative consent.

Enthusiastic consent implies that someone has voiced what they would like to do and asked the other party if they would like to do the same. It means that the individuals are approaching sex like a partnership instead of a "control over" situation. Although this shift in "scripts" may feel awkward for some initially, essentially it is just working on better, more power-balanced and clear communication.

Consent Is Specific

Consent to one activity doesn't mean that consent is given for another activity. Agreeing to go on a date with someone doesn't mean consent to have sex. Agreeing to go to someone's bedroom to kiss doesn't mean that you have agreed to have sex. Consent must be specific.

Parents can be very influential in shaping children's ability to experience healthy relationships and closeness with other people. From birth, babies desire closeness and bodily contact. Also from birth, parents send signals about what is appropriate and encouraged in terms of intimacy and expression. By starting early with the lifelong process, young people can be empowered with healthy values, skills, and information to foster positive, safe, and fulfilling relationships.

Consent and Technology

Another, newer layer necessary to explore when having conversations about consent is the role of technology and social media. An increasing number of young people report having been exposed to sexual content through various media platforms.

Young people today navigate different types of relationships than their parents did at that stage of development. Sexting, or sending and receiving sexual messages through technology like phones, emails, apps, or webcams, has become increasingly prevalent among young people and adults alike. Some find sexting to be the ultimate "safe sex" and a healthy way to explore sexuality that may or may not involve present or future physical contact. But it can also be used to bully, exploit, or even blackmail. And in some forms and dependent on age, it can be illegal.

Another layer to the complexity of consent with sexting is that even if someone consents initially to giving or receiving sex-related content, they may not be consenting to distribution of that content. "Revenge Porn" happens when someone shares someone else's private sex-related content with others as "payback." It can also additionally be used as a form of blackmail. Laws surrounding revenge porn vary.

In the case of both physical sexual contact and digital sexual contact, it is important that if people choose to engage in sexting it is done without pressure, manipulation, or false pretenses. Informed discussion about sexting can be beneficial in reducing both emotional and legal risk.

According to a recent survey from Kids Help Phone, about 28 percent of young people who sent sexual messages felt pressured into doing it.[27] Additionally, many apps provide opportunities for people to pose as someone they are not and it can sometimes be difficult to verify the authenticity of online users.

In addition to emotional and consent-related risks involved with sexting, there are also legal ramifications to consider. Young people and adults alike may not know that sexting can be illegal and can lead to criminal prosecution. Also, although it may be counterintuitive, the legal age of consent for sexual contact is often different from the legal age of consent for sexting (or development, distribution, duplication, or exchange of images of individuals involved in sexually explicit conduct). For example, in a state where the legal age of sexual consent is sixteen, the age at which it would be legal to send a nude photo of oneself without breaking the law could be eighteen.

Though laws vary from country to country and state to state, when sexting involves minors, it can violate both state and federal child pornography laws. Depending on the place, the government can prosecute individuals for production, distribution, reception, and possession of child pornography. Many states also have specific laws that address sexting specifically, with some having felony provisions for sexting that may result in required sex-offender registration, and more lenient states with provisions to treat it as a violation with a resulting fine, mandated counseling, or community service. Laws may also vary depending on whether the sending or receiving parties are minors who are close in age. Additionally, variance exists in sexting consent, with most state laws concluding that minors cannot provide consent to sext. It is important to understand what the laws are in your area (usually very easily found online with a simple search) before engaging with young people about the potential risks involved in sexting.

CHAPTER FIVE

··

Pornography and Sexting

Talking about the "Tough Stuff"

Never before have young people had greater access to digital messaging and imagery. A recent study conducted by Common Sense Media found that American adolescents consume an average of nine hours of media every day, which did not include the media that was used for work at school or home.[28] Within that consumption, they are exposed to many messages about sex and sexuality. Ideas about what sex should look like, what bodies should look like, how to get sex, and how to be sexual are shaped in part by these exposures. Young people and adults are exposed to messages about sexuality through billboards, radio, television, social media, electronic messaging, and video games on a nearly constant basis.

Some of the messaging that is consumed is positive and models healthy relationships and positive examples of sexual identities that we may not otherwise be exposed to. Media exposure can also be a tool to show how concepts like consent, sexual orientation, and gender identity are expressed in real life and can provide teaching opportunities for parents. Children who grow up feeling like they are different from their peers, in terms of sexual orientation or gender identity, may also find it comforting to see other people like them on television and in movies. Media exposure can be helpful in creating a sex-positive environment and cannot simply be reduced to being "good or bad." It is perhaps appropriate to view media exposure as consisting of both opportunity and risk.

Childhood Exposure to Pornography

It is reasonable to be interested in the impact of media exposure, or of anything we are exposed to for nine hours a day for that matter. Researchers are interested as well and explore the impact of media on physical, mental, and emotional health. One subset of this research focuses on the impact of exposure to pornography (sexually explicit material that is generally intended to arouse an audience). It is difficult to conduct "good research" exploring how pornography exposure impacts children because, as one could imagine, the ethical issues surrounding collecting that data are great. Some other limitations concerning discussing the impact of pornography exposure include:

- There is no one "type" of pornography. Forms (e.g., text, images, stories, anime, videos) and content (sexualities and behaviors represented) and production context (images taken consensually with relationships at home, images taken without consent, videos made through exploitation) vary considerably.

- Personal factors (age, ability to critically analyze material, access to "balancing factors" to counter messages received) likely impact the influence of exposure. People aren't consuming pornography in a vacuum. Individual, interpersonal, organizational, community, and policy factors are also shaping the way people process the information received. Differences in sexuality education and familial influence are great.

- Role of the consumer (passive consumption vs. active production). The impact for those consuming pornography passively may be different from the impact for those involved in producing pornography.

It is reasonable to be cautious about findings regarding the impacts of pornography exposure. However, one review of the literature examining the effects of pornography on children and young people summarized the ways in which environmental and social factors impact access and exposure to pornography among young people as described below.[29] The information was adapted from the "Socio-ecological context shaping access/exposure to online pornography" model.

Some factors that influence access and exposure to pornography and internet access in children and young people are:

Intrapersonal factors

- Age—Internet access increases as young people get older.

- Sex—Males are more likely to spend more time gaming and are more likely to deliberately seek out pornography and to do so frequently. Females are more likely to spend more time on social networking sites.

- Developmental maturity—Cognitive and psychological maturity impacts consumption of online pornography.

Techno sub-system factors

- Internet connection access—Children who grow up in homes with internet access are more likely to access greater amounts of online pornography.

- Number of devices in home—The number of devices may influence consumption.

- Mobile phone ownership—currently about two-third of twelve- and thirteen-year-olds own cell phones.

- Reasons that individuals access the web—Purposes for using internet vary (education, information seeking) and influence pornography access.

- Use of public and commercial hotspots—Access to hotspots can influence exposure.

Interpersonal factors

- Parental awareness—Parental knowledge of internet activity influences exposure and decreases as children get older.

- Peer use—The ways in which peers use the internet influence individual exposure.

Organizational/institutional factors

- Class standing—Internet and pornography consumption increases with the start of secondary school (high school).

- Age of educators—Many educators are now "digital natives" that have grown up with digital media exposure and are more likely to use the internet in classrooms and for assignments which may influence internet access among young people.

Community factors

- Perception of online risk—Experience with harm (cyberbullying, nonconsensual image distribution) may influence exposure.

- Spaces—The nature of links between online and offline spaces may influence exposure.

Socio-cultural factors

- Social inclusion—The normalization of the need for people to belong and connect through the internet increases the perceived importance of web use.

- Convergence—The convergence between different types of devices and media platforms influence web access.

Impact of Childhood Exposure to Pornography

There have been many researchers interested in examining the link between pornography exposure and sexual violence. No credible research to date has been able to assign a "causal" link between consumption of pornography and sexual-violence perpetration. This may be because it isn't linked or that we are limited in our ability to capture the link using current methodologies. It is important to consider the limitations of the research as described above. It is also important to examine the ways in which pornography can shape our ideas about gender, equality, sexuality, and intimate relationships as we consider its impact in direct and indirect ways. It may be appropriate to consider the cumulative effect of exposure in terms not only of its immediate impact but also of the impacts on society in a broader cultural context. It is also necessary to consider the role of "alternate narratives" and the ways we can effectively deconstruct the narratives often presented in pornography, especially when talking to young people.

While there are many limitations in the research, key findings presented in a 2017 extensive literature review found consistency in some findings about the influence of pornography consumption.[30] Key findings of their review are described below.

Knowledge, awareness, and education

- Pornography can educate consumers about sexual acts, practices, and diverse sexualities. Research indicates that porn can be main source of sexuality education if other explicit information is not available.

Attitudes, beliefs, and expectations about sex

- Adolescents' use of pornography is associated with stronger permissive attitudes including attitudes about casual and premarital sex.

- The types of behaviors and practices viewed through pornography can influence expectations about sex including expectations about what men find pleasurable and what people expect their partners to do. This may produce anxiety and fear.

- The gap between expectations and personal realities can produce "sexual uncertainty" about sexual beliefs and values and may increase the likelihood of sexual dissatisfaction.

Sexual behaviors and practices

- Some evidence suggests that exposure to pornography can increase the likelihood of earlier first-time sexual experience, particularly among adolescents who consume it regularly.

- Exposure to pornography can encourage young people to try acts viewed in dominant hetero pornography including anal intercourse, facial ejaculation, sex with multiple partners, and deep fellatio.

- Pornography exposure is also associated with unsafe behaviors including not using condoms and unsafe vaginal and anal sex.

Attitudes, beliefs, and expectations about gender

- Pornography may be associated with stronger beliefs in gender stereotypes. The association seems to be stronger for males.

- Male adolescents who view pornography frequently may be more likely to have sexist views.

- Some studies show a strengthening of existing attitudes supportive of violence against women and sexual violence with pornography exposure.

- Adolescent consumption of violent pornography is positively correlated with sexual aggression (though there are a variety of intersecting factors that may influence this correlation).

Mental health and well-being

- Exposure to pornography is associated with feelings of distress among younger children, particularly females (age nine to twelve).

- Exposure to pornography in adolescents may increase self-objectification and body surveillance.

Again, it is necessary to consider the limitations of the data gathering processes in considering the information above. It is also important to consider the countering factors that can influence the ways in which pornography exposure impacts individuals. In the absence of other countering measures and a solid, medically accurate sexuality education, the narratives created with pornography can be very influential in the formative years. But with a strong sexuality education and sex-positive guidance from parents and influential others, the impacts of pornography consumption may look drastically different. One of the key issues then may not just be the content and impact of pornography itself but also the absence of alternative narratives.

Suggestions for Discussing Pornography with Your Child

Countering messages and creating a safe environment in which kids can ask questions may be an effective way to provide alternative narratives about sexual attitudes and behaviors that may be shaped by pornography. Talking about pornography can feel daunting. Approaching discussions with a "media critical" (which can be universally applied to a variety of types of media exposures) lens may be helpful.

When helping people make sense of messages they are exposed to, it can helpful to consider:

- What is the purpose of the message? Is it to sell something? Who benefits?

- Who is delivering the message? Is the person engaged in the behavior the one who is actually making decisions about the content of the message? Is there a power imbalance? Who benefits?

- How does the message make you feel? Does exposure to the message make you feel better about yourself or worse? Does it make you feel frightened? Or pressured?

- What do you think is the intent of the message? What is being communicated?

- Is it realistic? Is it depicting the way things really are?

Using these approaches to examine all types of media (when watching commercials, examining online ads, watching television shows) can help to develop a critical lens in young people, which may be helpful as they navigate all types of digital messaging. Make these critical conversations a normalized part of discussions.

"Sexting" and Young People

"Sexting" is the sending and receiving of sexually explicit imagery through some form of digital messaging, usually through mobile phones. Although our understanding of the impacts of sexting is in its infancy, a few concerns that have emerged include:

- Images (particularly of young women) being distributed without consent

- Mobile phones being "vehicles" for the perpetration of sexual assault

- Social, legal, and psychological consequences experienced by people who are victimized by its distribution (exclusion from friend groups, moving schools, school suspension)

- Legal consequences with lifelong impacts for those who distribute (including risk of criminal charges for production and distribution of child pornography, mandated placement on sex-offender registries)

- The addition to broader cultural practices of sexualization, particularly among young women and adolescents

- Desensitization to sexually explicit imagery of young people

- The prevalence of coercion or pressure to send sexually explicit images

- "Revenge porn," or the distribution (or threat of distribution) of sexually explicit images as a way to enact revenge on another

Though attitudes vary among young people, many think of sending sexy messages or sending nude selfies as a way to flirt and express their sexuality. Due to their stage of brain development, it can also be difficult for adolescents to conceptualize the potential for long-term consequences that might be associated with sending or distributing sexually explicit images.

Having honest conversations with young people about potential consequences that may result from sexting as well as parental expectations concerning electronic devices can be helpful in influencing their decision-making process. One important component of that conversation should include the legal implications of sexting and distributing sexual images.

Though laws and legal consequences vary from country to country and state to state, it is currently illegal in the United States to "produce, distribute, receive, or possess with intent to distribute an obscene visual depiction of a minor (youth under the age of eighteen) engaged in sexually explicit conduct." Many states have specific laws that apply to sexting, minors sending, minors receiving, and individual "revenge porn" laws. You can find specific information about laws in your state on the following website: cyberbullying.org/sexting-laws. It is important to note that even in states with younger ages of consent for sexual activity, when it applies to sexual imagery, minors are considered those under the age of eighteen.

In addition to discussing potential legal consequences associated with sexting, it is important to discuss other components of the decision-making process. Encourage young people to think about whether sending sexual messages is something they want to do or if they are being pressured to do so. Pressure to move beyond sexual boundaries is a sign of an unhealthy relationship. It is also important to consider the likelihood that the message will get shared with others. If a phone is lost, stolen, or hacked, pictures can inadvertently be shared. Pictures can also be shared after a fight or breakup without the consent of the person sending it. It is almost impossible to guarantee the privacy of messages or pictures, and once it is sent, control of the message is transferred to the receiver.

What should children do if they receive an unsolicited sext or naked picture?

- Delete it as soon as possible.

- Talk to the sender about why sending it isn't a good idea. Consider other ways of flirting and expressing feelings.

- Do not show it to anyone. Sharing the picture, or even showing someone else, if the person is under eighteen is a crime.

- If you think someone is being bullied or harassed, talk to a trusted adult. In that case, it may be appropriate to save the photo to immediately show to a parent or other trusted adult.

Parental Monitoring of Digital Behavior

According to recent research from the Pew Research Center, 94 percent of thirteen to seventeen-year-olds own a desktop or laptop computer, 76 percent own a smartphone, 72 percent use Facebook, and 84 percent go online at least occasionally.[31] Constant parental monitoring is impossible, particularly in the older teenage years. Parents can take a number of different steps to monitor behavior in digital spaces. It is important to find a balance between respecting privacy and providing reasonable monitoring practices. Consider your own values and boundaries as you ponder approaches that feel appropriate in your home. Some considerations could include:

- Checking children's web-browsing history to note anything that might be concerning

- Reviewing children's friends on social media, especially for strangers who do not seem "age appropriate"

- Setting boundaries regarding time on social media and the internet, including time restrictions for using phones during nighttime hours

- Checking children's social media profiles. Become "friends" and follow them on Twitter

- Considering use of parental controls that block or filter content

- Limiting screen time

- Limiting the platforms that children can have access to

CHAPTER SIX

....

Sex, Virginity, and Sexual Response

The White, Black, and Gray Areas of Sex

Many things influenced my ideas about sex as a young person. I remember eagerly awaiting sex ed in the fifth grade. The buzz was palpable in the classrooms as all of us brought our signed permission slips, with a feeling that these were the tickets to get all our burning questions answered by the experts. Though each of us were too embarrassed to ask questions ourselves, we all sat in anticipation, hoping that some other kid would ask our burning question and it would then be answered out loud. But the "expert" for the "boy room" appeared to just be the only male teacher on staff, and the "expert" for the "girl room" was the female gym teacher everyone was afraid of—certainly too afraid of to ask questions about sex. And when the day finally came (yes, THE day, the single day), the take-away that most of us left with after watching the twenty-year-old film and sitting in silence for twenty minutes because nobody would ask questions, was that we were all going to get periods and armpit hair and that we should stay virgins for seemingly forever. I also remember talking about sex in my youth group at church, but the content of the conversations was almost exclusively again centered around the virtues of "virginity" (my reasoning for putting quotes around "virginity" will become clear).

I think it is fair to say that most parents want their children to remain abstinent while they are young. To reach that goal, it is necessary to understand the ways in which social and environmental influences shape sexual behavior choices. There are a complex variety of community, family, school, peer, relationship, and individual factors that interact to determine sexual behaviors in young people. Parental relationships and behaviors play an important role. Some family factors that are described as "protective" to either encourage abstinence or reduce the risk of early pregnancy and/or sexually transmitted disease include (adapted from Kirby and Lepore's report on Sexual Risk and Protective Factors):[32]

Protective family factors:

- A supportive, responsive parenting style

- A home environment that is oriented toward future goals

- Balanced parental monitoring

- Family connectedness

- Communication about sex, condoms, and contraception

- Communication about parental disapproval of sex in adolescence

- Higher family income and higher level of parental education

Family risk factors:

- Substance use in the household

- Over-controlling parenting styles

However, many methods currently used by schools, churches, and parents to encourage abstinence and risk avoidance are at best ineffective and at worst responsible for helping to create a harmful culture of shame that can have lifelong impacts.

"Virginity"

Shame-Based Tactics

The harmful tactics that promote abstinence and encourage "virginity" include the use of shame-based metaphors in sexuality-education curricula in schools and church programs. One of the frequently used examples is that of "The Tape." In this demonstration a child, usually a teenage boy, is called to come to the front of the class and "have sex with his girlfriend" (represented by sticking a piece of tape to his arm). The couple then "breaks up" (demonstrated by ripping the tape off of his arm). The used piece of tape now has hair, skin cells, oil, and lotion on it and has lost some of its adhesive. Next, the instructor asks another student (almost always male) to come forward and "have sex with the ex-girlfriend" (demonstrated by applying the used tape to the new volunteer's arm). After their certain breakup (tearing of the tape off the arm) and the same demonstration with a few other boys, the class sees that the tape now has lost all of its adhesive (its sole purpose as a piece of tape) and is dirty and full of cologne, hair, dirt, lotion, oil, and skin cells. The visual is often accompanied with the message that sex decreases our ability to bond with others and somehow indirectly changes our value and desirability to partners.

Another popular shame-based metaphor that is frequently used is "The Spit Cup." In this demonstration, an instructor starts with clean glasses of water and asks several students, again usually male, to take a drink and then swish it around their mouths (representing sex) and then spit all the water back into a glass. But now instead of the water being clean, it is full of food particles and is no longer clean. Then the instructor holds up a clean, clear class of water in one hand, and a murky, spit-filled glass of water in the other and says, "which one would you want to date?" Still other metaphors used all over the country compare having had sex with multiple partners as being like a "rose with all its petals plucked off" or like a "chewed piece of gum."

In a speech given by Elizabeth Smart in 2014, she described being kidnapped, raped, and held in captivity as a child. She recalled a lesson that she learned in school about having sex before marriage:

"For me, I thought, 'Oh my gosh. I'm that chewed up piece of gum. Nobody re-chews a piece of gum. You throw it away.' And that's how easy it is to feel like you no longer have worth, you no longer have value. Why would it even be worth screaming out? Why would it even make a difference if you are rescued, if your life still has no value?"

In these shaming metaphors, people who have sex are almost always presented as tarnished and worthless. And often the target is female. In the situations in which girls engage in sexual behavior (either by choice or by force) the label that follows often carries unique and overstated generalizations about moral character. There are many reasons that abstinence can improve health outcomes for young people, but trying to promote abstinence through the use of shaming metaphors can have long-lasting negative emotional and physical impacts. These messages can also be particularly harmful for those who have experienced sexual abuse and may be having sex without consent. Attaching personal value to sexuality is problematic in a variety of ways.

One danger in overemphasizing the value of "virginity" (in most examples, it's female "virginity") is that it devalues the other aspects of the complete self, sending cues that female sexuality is the apex of desirability to a partner. The value of the intellectual self, the capable self, the holistic self, is conversely understated in terms of gifts that females can bring to relationships. The danger of this messaging exists not only in its narrowly defined suitability to potential mates but also in how it inadvertently (ironically) objectifies and hypersexualizes girls and women.

Elevating "virginity" as a marker of worth can also put young people at physical risk by decreasing their likelihood of reporting sexual assault and rape. Additionally, attaching sex with feelings of shame can interfere with lifelong sexual satisfaction and health.

"Sex" Means Different Things to Different People

"I did not have sexual relations with that woman, Ms. Lewinsky." Most will remember this statement from President Clinton in 1998, as he denied having an affair with former intern Monica Lewinsky. During a later deposition meant to determine whether he'd committed perjury with that statement, he was asked to clarify if the sexual acts that he engaged in met the definition of "sexual relations" as presented by the Independent Counsel's Office. He later clarified that it was his belief that he had not engaged in sexual relations as defined, because he had not come into contact with the body parts described in the stated definition and had only received oral sex and not given it.

This confusion highlights some of the disagreement that exists just in defining the act of "sex." Is oral sex, sex? Is giving it sex but receiving it isn't? Is it only sex if it can result in pregnancy? If so, does that mean people who only engage in same-sex behavior stay virgins forever? Is anal sex, sex? Is receiving it sex but giving it isn't? Is it only sex if the hymen is disrupted? Sex means different things to different people.

The concept of virginity is socially constructed, meaning that we create, assign, and accept an idea or definition based on collected views within a society. If sex means different things to different people, then virginity does as well. This can be problematic, as some educational programs and conversations emphasize virginity and abstinence, even though these terms are subjective. This may encourage people to engage in risky behavior, believing that they are still "virgins" if they are engaging in same-sex sexual behavior or other activities that are not penile-vaginal sex, including oral or anal sex. For these reasons, it is important to use plain language that focuses on *behaviors* and not *socially constructed labels* when talking to young people about sexuality.

Types of Sexual Activity

There are many ways in which people can engage in sexual activity and receive sexual pleasure. This list is by no means exhaustive:

Kissing—Kissing is a form of romantic or sexual expression in which lips are pressed against the lips of another. It may also include "French kissing" where the tongue is inserted into the mouth of another.

Massage and erotic massage—Massage is rubbing the body of another to create tension release and pleasure. Erotic massage can be performed to elicit sexual pleasure and usually involves contact with sexual anatomy. Both can be done with oils or lotions.

"Sexting" or phone sex—Sexting is sending, receiving, or forwarding sexually explicit messages through cell phones or through another digital device. This can also include talking on the phone with someone while masturbating or exchanging fantasies and sexual content.

Cunnilingus (oral sex of the vulva)—Cunnilingus involves stimulation of the vulva, vagina, and clitoris by the mouth, lips, and tongue of another. It can be for the purpose of foreplay or as a complete sexual act.

Fellatio (oral sex of the penis and testicles)—Fellatio involves the oral stimulation of the penis and scrotum (using the lips, tongue, mouth, and throat, in what is sometimes described as "teabagging"). Fellatio may involve ingestion of semen or not.

Analingus ("rimming")—Analingus is a type of oral sex in which a person orally stimulates the anus with the mouth, lips, and tongue. If performed without a dental dam, health risks can include a transmission of a variety of fecal-orally transmitted infections, including E. coli, forms of hepatitis, and other conditions.

Group sex—Group sex is sexual behavior that involves more than two participants.

Solo masturbation—Solo masturbation involves the personal manual stimulation or stimulation with toys of the penis, vulva, vagina, clitoris, or anus to achieve sexual pleasure. Masturbation can be a good way for people to get to know their body and what they like. Although there are many myths about masturbation, there is no credible scientific evidence that indicates that masturbation will cause any physical or mental health problems when proper hygiene is observed. Proper masturbation hygiene includes:

- Washing hands before and after touching the penis, vulva, vagina, clitoris, or anus

- Cleaning sex toys/masturbation tools with every use to reduce the risk of infection

- Using a condom on sex toys if they are passed between partners, and changing the condom so it is only used by one person

- Wash sex toys/masturbation tools after using them in the anus, particularly before moving to another body part

Mutual masturbation/Manual sex—Typically involves manual stimulation of the genitals by two or more people who stimulate themselves or each other. It can be used as a form of foreplay or as a primary sexual activity. When performing a "hand job" the penis or scrotum are manually stimulated. In fingering, the vagina, clitoris, or other parts of the vulva are manually stimulated. Fingering may also include simulation of the anus.

Mammary intercourse—This sexual activity is performed by placing the penis in between the breasts of another and moving the penis up and down to mimic penetration.

"Dry humping" or frottage—"Dry humping" is sexual activity that usually does not include penetration and may include kissing, cuddling, and mutual masturbation. Frottage is the term used to describe rubbing any part of the body of another person whether clothed or unclothed.

Tribadism—Tribadism or "scissoring" is a form of sexual activity where women rub genitalia against each other, either together or on other parts of the body.

Penile-vaginal intercourse—Penile-vaginal intercourse involves inserting and thrusting the penis into the vagina for sexual pleasure or reproduction.

Anal intercourse—Anal intercourse is the insertion and thrusting of the penis into a person's anus for sexual pleasure. This activity can occur in same-sex and other-sex relationships.

BDSM (Bondage, Discipline, (or domination), Sadism, and Masochism)— This sexual activity involves the use of physical restraints, granting and relinquishing control, and the inflection of pain for sexual pleasure. BDSM is evolved into a "catch-all" phrase that covers a wide range of activities, interpersonal relationships, and distinct subcultures. Different from domestic violence, it involves informed consent between participants (the dominant and submissive partners) and may even involve written contracts, "safe words" that indicate when approaching or crossing, a physical, emotional, or moral boundary, that typically involve discussion and negotiation in advance of engaging in behaviors.

Unique Sexual Concerns among the LGBTQ+ Population

LGBTQ+ youth need and deserve to learn in settings that are inclusive of their experiences and that give them the education necessary to stay safe and healthy. Most teens who have been surveyed state that they have not had sexuality education that covered same-sex relationships.[33] Individuals who identify as LGBTQ+ may have unique concerns regarding sexuality that are often not addressed in school sexuality-education programs that focus largely on pregnancy prevention. Programs that are solely based on pregnancy prevention often leave out content that can be helpful in keeping safe those who do not identify as heterosexual.

According to recent CDC data concerning adults and teens:[34]

- Adult and adolescent gay and bisexual men made up 70 percent of new HIV infections

- MSM (men who have sex with men) make up 58 percent of new cases of syphilis

- Bacterial Vaginosis is more common among women who have sex with women (WSW)

- The pregnancy rate for lesbian and bisexual women in their teens are two to seven times greater than their straight peers

In addition to limited sexuality education in schools, a recent study conducted by Planned Parenthood revealed that LGBTQ+ youth have a limited number of trusted adults they feel comfortable talking about sexual health with, so much information is attained from less than ideal sources.[35]

Inclusive discussions about sexuality should happen in the home and in school and should include the following, which adapted from information provided by SIECUS:[36]

- Information about a broad spectrum of sexual orientations including age-appropriate and medically accurate information

- Information about a broad spectrum of gender identities including age-appropriate and medically accurate information

- Positive examples of individuals who identify LGBTQ+ in course content

- Examples of individuals who identify as LGBTQ+ within the context of romantic relationships, sexual relationships, and families

- Discussion about staying safe and the need for protection during sex for people of all identities

- Discussion of myths and stereotypes about behavior and identity

Sex among Those with Disabilities

Physical and mental disabilities can impact sexuality in direct and indirect ways. People with disabilities can also erroneously be viewed as asexual when this is often not the case. Because of this perception, people with disabilities are often left out of sexuality education and are at increased risk for sexual assault and abuse and other negative outcomes. According to a recent study looking at sexual activity in young adults with and without mild/moderate disability, "most young people with mild/moderate intellectual disabilities have had sexual intercourse by age nineteen or twenty, although young women were less likely to have sex prior to sixteen than their peers and both men and women with intellectual disabilities were more likely to have unsafe sex 50 percent or more of the time than their peers."[37] Teenagers with disabilities often have inadequate knowledge about contraception and disease prevention. People who suffer from attention deficit disorders may also struggle to achieve intimacy with others without exposure to specialized skills training.

Parents and schools can work together to foster behavioral and cognitive change that can help people with developmental disabilities manage their sexual needs in ways that are healthy and appropriate. People with disabilities have a right to express their sexuality and deserve access to information to help keep them safe. People with intellectual and developmental disabilities may need specialized approaches to sexuality education, including education in how to manage sexuality in private, including solo sex. They may also need specialized approaches to learning about and using birth control.

Among those with developmental disabilities that limit or change sexual function, specialized education and skills training can also be appropriate to foster healthy sexual expression. Those with spinal cord injuries may have challenges regarding sexual response but can often experience some level of satisfying sexual functioning. It is important to refrain from making assumptions about asexuality or a lack of sexual interest among those with disabilities and facilitate individualized access to sexuality education and birth control if appropriate.

Sexual Response–What Happens in the Body during Sex?

Although many factors influence how people experience sex (including our thoughts about our own bodies, our perceptions about the morality of sexual activity, parental relationships, fear of sexual activity and vulnerability, and having a history of abuse), from a physiological perspective, there are typically fairly predictable processes that happen in the body in response to sexual arousal.

There are many similarities between all genders in terms of physiological response to sexual stimulation. Researchers describe the sequence of physical reactions that occur in the body in response to sexually stimulating activities (including masturbation) as the sexual response cycle. It is important to note that although the sexual response cycle includes orgasm and resolution, not all sexual stimulation results in orgasm. Many people who do not reach orgasm can still find sexual stimulation to be satisfying. There are other models used to describe this process with some variation, but this four-phase model captures the key elements of the response process.

Sexual Response Cycle (adapted from Masters and Johnson's model of Sexual Response)[38]

Excitement—As a person becomes sexually aroused, the following changes may occur:

- Muscular tension, heart rate, and blood pressure increases

- Skin may become flushed with blotches appearing on the chest and back

- Blood flow to the genitals increases, resulting in swelling of clitoris in females (f) and erection of the penis in males (m)

- Nipples become erect; breasts become fuller (f)

- The vagina lubricates, expands, becomes darker in color, and lengthens (f)

- Testicles swell, scrotum tightens and thickens, and urethral diameter begins to widen (m)

Plateau—This phase follows excitement and continues to the brink of orgasm and includes:

- Muscular tension, heart rate, and blood pressure continue to increase

- Nipples become turgid

- Sex flush appears in most and begins to spread

- Clitoris retracts under the foreskin and becomes increasingly sensitive (f)

- Vagina expands more and lengthens, forms the "orgasmic platform" (swollen tissue that reduces the diameter of the vaginal opening, in which contractions occur during orgasm) (f)

- The uterus becomes fully elevated in the body (f)

- Labia swell more and become darker in color (f)

- Penis increases in diameter and becomes fully erect (m)

- Testes enlarge and elevate toward the body (m)

- The Cowper's gland releases a few drops of fluid ("precum") (m)

Orgasm—This phase signifies climax and is typically the shortest phase of the cycle and is present if sexual activity results in an orgasm. It may include:

- Blood pressure, respiration, and heart rate reach peak intensity

- Sex flush deepens

- Loss of voluntary muscle control and spasms in some muscles

- Sudden, forceful release of sexual tension

- Uterus engages in wavelike contractions, the muscles of the vagina contract (f)

- Penis and urethra undergo contractions that release semen (m)

Resolution—In this phase, the body returns to its unaroused state.

- Respiration, heart rate, and blood pressure return to normal

- Sex flush disappears

- Film of perspiration may appear on the skin

- Muscles relax

- Labia return to unaroused size, position, and color (f)

- Uterus lowers to normal position (f)

- The opening of the cervix of the uterus widens for twenty to thirty minutes (f)

- Vaginal walls relax and return to unaroused color (f)

- Penis loses its erection (m)

- Scrotal skin relaxes and thins to unaroused state (m)

- Testes return to unaroused size and position (m)

- Refractory period of varying length present, in which one cannot be restimulated to orgasm (m)

How to Know When You Are Ready for Sex

Young people (and not-so-young people) are naturally curious about how they will know when it is right to engage in sexual activity with another person. It is important for parents and young people to understand the laws surrounding sexual activity (including sexual activity over digital devices). It is also important for parents to clearly state their expectations regarding sexual behavior. Parental expectations are an important factor in young people's decision-making processing.

Sex feels good. And when we try to hide that from young people and only talk about the negative aspects of sexuality it comes out as disingenuous, as it contradicts nearly everything else they hear. The disconnect may also add to the "mysticism" that may inadvertently encourage exploration. When all conversations about sex are focused on infections, unplanned pregnancy, and consent/sexual assault issues, it can also create unnecessary anxieties and an incomplete and potentially harmful view of sexuality. Additionally, it makes parents and other "trusted adults" appear deceptive and potentially undesirable sources of accurate information about sex. If the goal is to be a resource for kids, lead with honesty.

Having balanced conversations about the risks and benefits of intimate relationships from a "sex-positive" framework can minimize shame and foster healthier perceptions about sexuality. Emphasizing that sex and sexual pleasure are normal components of healthy, adult, consensual relationships and that sex helps people to connect and make each other feel good is a great place to start.

Young people (and not-so-young people) may also have a lot of questions about how a person knows they are ready to have sex with someone. Discussing potential considerations may help with the decision-making process.

Things to consider before having sex:

- How do you feel about the other person? Are you trying to use sex to make them like you more or because you feel ready?

- Am I using sex to provide validation? Do I feel a personal sense of value without sex?

- Do you understand that sex doesn't "make someone love you" or make them stay with you?

- Have you discussed what you are and are not willing to do sexually with your partner?

- Have you talked about expectations of privacy (who, if anyone, you are comfortable knowing that you have been intimate)?

- Can you describe your boundaries and know that they will be respected?

- Do you agree on what "sex" means? Different partners may have different ideas about what sex is, and it is important to make sure they understand what they are agreeing to.

- How do you think you will feel after?

- Have you discussed sexual histories? If you or the other person have had sex before, it is a good idea to get tested for STIs.

- Can you agree to stop midway or right before if you change your mind or are feeling uncomfortable?

- Is sex with the other person legal according to the laws in my state? (See Chapter Four for more on consent and legal issues.)

- Am I comfortable speaking with a medical professional about birth control, STI testing, and questions regarding sexual health care needs?

- Am I comfortable and able to describe my sexual needs and desires with my partner? Are they comfortable describing theirs to me?

- Are you able to be intimate with the person with a clear head? Do you need alcohol, drugs, or other substances in order to feel like you are "ready" or interested?

- Do the behaviors that you are considering align with your values and your goals for your future?

CHAPTER SEVEN

....

Making Sex Safer

Staying Safe When Choosing to Be Sexually Active

Many parents, understandably, have a hard time imagining their children eventually becoming sexually active beings. Because of this, some may find it unnecessary to discuss topics related to practicing safer sex. Research suggests that about 97 percent of adults report ever having engaged in sexual contact, so it is reasonable to assume that, even if your child isn't having sex now, they eventually will become sexually active. Many models of sex-education curricula in schools emphasize abstinence and provide very little information about staying safe if young people decide to become sexually active. Because young people are exposed to frequent examples of unsafe sex practices and so much misinformation exists about sex safety, parents may find it helpful to be a resource for information on this topic.

Consistent data indicates that parents tend to be overly optimistic about their children's risk behaviors, underestimating the frequency of their children's alcohol, smoking, marijuana, and sex-related behaviors. Many young people engage in sexual behaviors that could result in pregnancy, sexually transmitted infection, and other unintended consequences. According to data from the 2017 Centers for Disease Control and Prevention report, of US high school students surveyed[39]

- 40 percent had ever had sexual intercourse

- 10 percent had four or more sexual partners

- 7 percent had been physically forced to have intercourse when they did not want to

- 30 percent had had sexual intercourse during the three previous months, and of these

  ◊ 46 percent did not use a condom the last time they had sex

  ◊ 14 percent did not use any method to prevent pregnancy

  ◊ 19 percent had drunk alcohol or used drugs before the last sexual intercourse

- Less than 10 percent of all students have ever been tested for HIV

Several factors may increase the likelihood of young people engaging in sexual risk behaviors. According to the data from the CDC, lesbian, gay, and bisexual high school students are more likely than their peers to be at risk of serious health outcomes. Sexual minority youth (defined as youth who identify as gay, lesbian, bisexual, and those who are not sure of their sexual identity) are more at risk of violence, HIV infection, STIs, and pregnancy. They also may encounter more issues with stigma, discrimination, social rejection, and family disapproval. Many models of school-based sexuality-education curricula also focus exclusively on heterosexual content.

Research also suggests that substance use can increase the likelihood of engaging in sexual risk behaviors. These risks include ever having sex, having multiple sex partners, not using a condom when having sex, and pregnancy before the age of fifteen. Substance use and sexual encounters and number of partners also seem to be positively correlated, meaning as substance use increases the likelihood in young people engaging in sex and the number of partners increase as well. According to the 2017 National Youth Risk Behavior Survey, of students who are currently sexually active, 19 percent drank alcohol or used drugs before their last sexual encounter.[40]

Although abstaining from oral, anal, and vaginal intercourse is the only "fool proof" way to prevent pregnancy and the spread of STIs, learning safer sex practices can dramatically reduce many of the health risks associated with sexual activity. It makes sense then that effective discussions about sexuality should include how to engage (at some point) in the safest and most satisfying practices possible to minimize unintended consequences.

Environmental factors and parental behaviors can play an important role in influencing substance use and sexual risk behaviors among young people. According to the CDC, common risk factors for substance use and sexual risk behaviors include:

- Extreme economic deprivation (poverty, over-crowding)
- Family history of the problem behavior, family conflict, and family management problems
- Favorable parental attitudes toward the problem behavior
- Parental involvement in the problem behavior
- Lack of positive parental engagement
- Association with substance-using peers
- Alienation and rebelliousness
- Lack of school connectedness

It may be helpful for parents to recognize personal risk factors that may apply to their children and to learn to communicate strategies that decrease unintended sexual risk among those young people who choose to be sexually active.

Barriers to Safe Sex Practices

One barrier that may inhibit young people from engaging in safer sexual practices is simply the lack of knowledge of how to do so. Although many leaders and parents erroneously believe that talking about safer sex and providing access to information and services related to sexual and reproductive health increases sexual behavior, there is strong scientific consensus that that simply is not true.

Parents may fear that having discussions about safer sex methods will reduce the perceived negative consequences of sexual behavior and may encourage young people to initiate sex or promote "promiscuity." However, a large body of evidence supports a comprehensive approach to sexuality education and risk reduction. A recent United Nations-commissioned review of twenty-two systematic studies suggested that comprehensive sex-education programs were associated with "delayed initiation of sexual intercourse, decreased frequency of sexual intercourse, fewer sexual partners, and less risk taking."[41] It follows that young people can only benefit from evidence-based information about sexual safety. However, many school sex-education programs are aimed at preventing sex and do not address concerns of youth who are already engaging in sexual behaviors, and do not teach safe sex practices, condom use, or other birth control methods. Many also leave out content that may specifically apply to youth who identify as part of the LGBTQ+ population.

Sexual Behavior and Health Risks

Many sexual behaviors carry some degree of health risk. While healthy expression of sexuality can add to physical, emotional, and mental health, sexual behavior also can carry varying levels of risks in terms of health outcomes.

Oral Sex

Oral sex involves contact of the mouth, lips, and tongue with the vulva and vaginal area (cunnilingus) or the mouth, lips, and tongue with the penis (fellatio) and the mouth, lips, and tongue with the anus (analingus or "rimming"). Although many young people don't even consider oral sex to be "sex," many STIs and other infections can be spread through oral sex. The level of risk for contracting an STI through oral sex depends on the particular STI, the prevalence of the STI in the community, and the number of sexual encounters. Oral sex poses health risks to the person performing the act and the person receiving it. Infection can occur in the mouth and throat, as well as in the vagina, penis, anus, or rectum. Some STIs (like syphilis, gonorrhea, and intestinal infections) can also be transmitted through oral sex and can then spread throughout the body. Some diseases that can be transmitted through oral sex include chlamydia, gonorrhea, syphilis, herpes, human papillomavirus (HPV), and HIV (low risk). Orally stimulating the anus can also transmit hepatitis A and B, intestinal parasites, and bacterial infections like E. coli.

Vaginal and Anal Sex

Vaginal sex, sometimes called penetrative vaginal sex, is when the penis is inserted into the vagina. Infections can be passed through vaginal fluids, blood, semen, skin to skin contact, or contact with mucous membranes. Infection can occur in both the penetrative and receptive partners.

Anal sex involves inserting the penis into the anus. Because of the thin tissue and the fact that the anus lacks the natural lubrication that the vagina provides, risk of tissue tears and disease transmission during unprotect penetration are high. Additionally, there is also a high likelihood that bacteria is present in the anus.

Some infections that can be passed through vaginal and anal sex include chlamydia, gonorrhea, hepatitis B, herpes, HIV, human papillomavirus (HPV), pubic lice, scabies, syphilis, trichomoniasis, and pelvic inflammatory disease.

Manual Sex

Manual sex (also called digital sex) is sexual activity that is performed with the hands. It can include sexual contact with the hand and fingers and the vulva and vaginal area, the penis, and the anus. Some may refer to it as a "hand job" or "fingering" or "fingerbanging." Though transmission is less likely than with vaginal and anal sex, unprotected manual stimulation can spread skin to skin infections for both partners, including herpes.

HIV and Young People

According to the CDC, an estimated 50,900 youth had HIV in 2016, and of those, only about 56 percent were aware of their infection.[42] Youth are the least likely of all age groups to be aware of their HIV status. Black males are at an increased risk, making up more than half of all new cases in young gay and bisexual men. The majority of new HIV diagnoses in youth occur through male to male sexual contact in men (93 percent), and heterosexual contact in females (86 percent). Although condoms are effective at significantly reducing the risk of transmitting HIV, as well as preventing many other sexually transmitted infections and pregnancy, many youths lack proper education in using them correctly and lack access to them. Both factors can contribute significantly to the likelihood of not using condoms and to the increase of common mistakes associated with improper use.

Proper Condom Use

External condoms are used to prevent pregnancy and protect against the transmission of STIs. They are made from a thin layer of latex, polyurethane, polyisoprene, or natural membrane and are worn over the penis during sexual contact. They can also be cut and placed over the vulva when performing oral sex on a female.

When reading about the efficacy of any birth control method, you will likely see two different numbers: "perfect use" and "typical use." Perfect use refers to the efficacy at preventing pregnancy if one hundred women were to use that method for a year in a theoretical or "perfect" scenario. Typical use is the same calculation, but factoring in how the method is typically used and considering human error. For example, when used to prevent pregnancy, it is often stated that male condoms have a perfect use failure rate of 2 percent. But the typical failure rate is much higher at about 15 percent. People often underestimate how complicated condom use can be. This discrepancy is due in part to these common errors:

- Not keeping condoms on throughout sexual intercourse

- Neglecting to leave space at the tip of the condom for ejaculate

- Putting the condom on inside out

- Not using appropriate lubricant

- Incorrect withdrawal of the penis

- Not squeezing air from the tip

It perhaps is not enough to tell sexually active people to use condoms, but also *how* to use them.

How to Use an External (Sometimes Referred to as a Male) Condom

If used correctly every single time, condoms are quite effective at preventing pregnancy and reducing the transmission of many sexually transmitted infections. The better that people are at using them correctly, the better they work! Some key factors that make condom use more effective are described below:

Timing: Condoms should be used every time an individual has vaginal, anal, and oral sex. Additionally, the condom should be worn from the beginning of the sexual experience (before the mouth, genital area, anus have experienced contact) to the end.

Ensure safe storage of condoms: Condoms can lose efficacy if not stored properly. Make sure condoms are kept away from heat, cold, and friction. Glove boxes in the car, freezers, wallets, etc. are inappropriate storage receptacles for those reasons. They should be kept in a cool dry place and away from sharp items or sunlight.

Check expiration date: Condoms that have expired are less effective. There should be an expiration date on the box of condoms and on the individual wrapper.

Visually inspect the condom: Take a close look at the condom to ensure that there are no tears or defects before placing it on the penis.

Roll the condom on the penis correctly: The condom should be placed on the penis while it is erect. Also, condoms will roll down the penis more effectively if they are placed on the penis the appropriate way. The "rim" of the condom should be placed as if it were a little hat (I tell my students it should look like a sombrero and not like a mushroom). It should roll down fairly easily if placed correctly on the penis.

Pinch the tip of the condom before placing it on the penis to allow for space at the tip: Leave enough room at the top of the condom for the semen to have space to be collected. The reduces the risk of it spilling out of the condom. For some who are uncircumcised, it may be more comfortable to first push back the foreskin before placing the condom on the penis.

Cover as much skin as possible: It is important to roll the condom to the base of the penis. Condoms provide protection not only by catching fluids passed during intercourse, but also by reducing the risk of infections caused by skin to skin contact. Increasing the amount of skin covered improves efficacy.

Use appropriate lube if desired: It can be helpful to place a few drops of water-based lubrication to the inside tip of a condom before rolling it on. Placing lubrication on the outside of the condom can also decrease the risk of condoms breaking. Use only water-based or silicone lubricants. Do not use Vaseline, petroleum jelly, cooking oils, butter, hand creams, body lotion. Those products can break down the condom and reduce their efficacy and increase the likelihood of breakage.

Use care when removing the condom: After ejaculation and while the penis is still erect, hold on firmly to the base of condom while removing the penis from the vagina, anus, or mouth. Be careful not to spill semen while removing the penis. Throw the condom in the garbage and do not dispose in the toilet as it will cause plumbing issues.

Remember that condoms are intended for single use: Do not reuse condoms. Use a new condom every time you engage in vaginal, oral, or anal sex or are switching between those modes (as in moving from anal sex to vaginal sex).

Sexual Activity and Risk

High-risk sexual activities:

- Sexual contact when blisters, sores, rashes, or abnormal discharge are present
- Sexual contact while under the influence of drugs or alcohol, which can increase the likelihood of engaging in high-risk activity
- Oral sex without the protection of a condom or dental dam
- Anal sex without proper condom use (the lining of the anus is much thinner than other tissues and can be easily damaged which can increase the spread of infection)
- Vaginal sex without proper condom use
- Using unclean sex toys or using with multiple partners
- Engaging in sexual activity with multiple partners
- Engaging in sexual activity with partners who are not monogamous
- Engaging in sexual activity with partners who inject drugs
- Oral sexual contact with oral ulcers, bleeding gums, or the presence of other STIs

Reducing risk:

- Practice abstinence (abstaining from oral, vaginal, and anal sex).

- Use a condom or dental dam correctly with each oral, vaginal, or anal sexual encounter.

- Use a finger cot (condom-like cover used over the finger or sex toys) during stimulation of the vulva, vagina, and clitoris.

- Use latex or polyurethane gloves during manual sex to increase safety.

- Get vaccinated to protect against human papillomavirus (HPV) (comes in a series of three vaccinations and will provide protection against cervical and other types of cancer).

- Get vaccinated to protect against hepatitis A and B (the mouth can come into contact with feces or other fluids that carry hepatitis during oral sex).

- Limit the number of sex partners.

- Talk to a doctor about pre-exposure prophylaxis (PrEP) if at very high risk for HIV.

- Practice good hygiene and keep genitals clean, including gently pulling back foreskin (if present) to clean the area that can harbor dead skin and secretions that may increase likelihood of transmitting infection.

- Avoid sexual contact if blisters, sores, or rashes are present on the genitals, anus, or mouth.

- Do not engage in sexual contact if under the influence of drugs or alcohol.

- Wash sex toys thoroughly after every use, when changing use (as in switching from anal use to vaginal use), and if switching between partners.

- Urinate after having sex to help prevent urinary tract infections.

- Refrain from vaginal "douching," which has been associated with various health concerns including increasing risk of infection like bacterial vaginosis.

- Get screened regularly for sexually transmitted infections (about every year or more if having sex with new partners).

- Use water-based lubricant with condoms to reduce the risk of breakage.

Female condoms can be used to reduce the risk of pregnancy and the transmission of sexually transmitted infections. They are made from a synthetic latex and are inserted into the vagina as far up as it will go. The ring rests against the cervix and expands after placement. Once firmly in place, the rest of the condom covers the vaginal canal and some of the external vulva area. They are more expensive and less available than male condoms.

Getting Tested

Regular testing is an important part of making sex safer and maintaining good health in people who are sexually active.

The CDC recommends the following regarding STD testing:[43]

- *All adults and adolescents from ages thirteen to sixty-four* should be tested at least once for HIV.

- *All sexually active women* younger than twenty-five years should be tested for gonorrhea and chlamydia every year. Women twenty-five years and older with risk factors such as new or multiple sex partners or a sex partner who has an STI should also be tested for gonorrhea and chlamydia every year.

- *All pregnant women* should be tested for syphilis, HIV, and hepatitis B starting early in pregnancy. At-risk pregnant women should also be tested for chlamydia and gonorrhea starting early in pregnancy. Testing should be repeated as needed to protect the health of mothers and their infants.

- *All sexually active gay and bisexual men* should be tested at least once a year for syphilis, chlamydia, and gonorrhea. Those who have multiple or anonymous partners should be tested more frequently for STIs (i.e., at three to six-month intervals).

- *Sexually active gay and bisexual men* may benefit from more frequent HIV testing (e.g., every three to six months).

- *Anyone who has unsafe sex or shares injection drug equipment* should get tested for HIV at least once a year.

CHAPTER EIGHT

....

Sexually Transmitted Infections

Facts, Not Fear

Because sexual activity allows for close bodily contact, the rubbing of warm, wet skin, and possibly the exchange of body fluids, it provides a likely pathway for the transmission of disease. Sexually transmitted infections are a serious public health concern, and, according to the CDC, fifteen to twenty-four-year-olds account for half of all sexually transmitted infections. Gay, bisexual, and other men who have sex with men (MSM) are also at an increased risk of STIs in the throat and rectum. Although they impact and affect people of all ages and socioeconomic statuses, they take a disproportionate toll on young people. At the time of this publication, the rate of STIs has surged for the fifth straight year and has reached an all-time high.

According to the CDC, there are currently:[44]

- 1.8 million cases of chlamydia, with a *19 percent increase* since 2014

- 583,405 cases of gonorrhea, with a *63 percent rate increase* since 2014

- 115,045 cases of syphilis, with a *71 percent rate increase* of infectious syphilis since 2014

- 1,306 cases of syphilis among newborns, with a *185 percent rate increase* since 2014

If left untreated, sexually transmitted infections can cause long-term problems including an increased risk of getting HIV if exposed and an increased risk of transmitting HIV if present, long-term pelvic/abdominal pain, an inability to get pregnant, and an increased risk of pregnancy complications.

If Someone Suspects They Have a Sexually Transmitted Infection

The most important first step to take if someone believes they may have contracted a sexually transmitted infection is to get tested. While many sexually transmitted infections have no symptoms, they can cause long-term complications if left untreated. Therefore, it is important to find out right away to start treatment. Many STIs are curable and treatable. People can access testing through their regular health care provider, local health care departments, family planning clinics, and urgent care providers.

Next, it is important to notify partners. Partner notification can protect their health by allowing them to get tested and potentially treated right away. Untreated STIs like gonorrhea and chlamydia can result in serious health complications like pelvic inflammatory disease, infertility, and potentially deadly ectopic pregnancies. Additionally, if STIs are left untreated, they can be passed back to the treated partner.

It is therefore important to get retested. People can get reinfected with the same sexually transmitted infection. Some strains of infection can also be resistant to certain treatments. It is important to get retested in three months, even if each partner was treated with medication.

How Are Sexually Transmitted Infections Spread?

Sexually transmitted infections can be spread through skin to skin contact, oral sex, vaginal-penile sex, and anal sex.

Skin to Skin Contact

An uninfected person doesn't necessarily have to have a cut in the skin to get an STI from an infected partner, although the likelihood of transmission goes up when cuts or open sores are present. Many STIs can be transmitted through mucus membranes of the mouth, lips, nostrils, eyelids, ears, anus, and parts of the genitals. Infection happens when a persons infected shedding skin cells, open lesions, body fluids, or mucous membranes come into contact with an uninfected person's mucous membranes or open lesions.

STIs that can be transmitted by skin to skin contact include type one and type two herpes, HPV, and syphilis. These are transmitted when an infected site of one individual's skin come into direct contact with a mucous membrane or lesion on an infected person.

Risks of skin to skin transmission in sexual contact can be reduced by avoiding sexual contact when herpes flare-ups are occurring, getting tested, encouraging sexual partners to get tested, using barriers like condoms and dental dams during sexual contact, getting vaccinated for HPV, and taking antiviral medication for herpes.

Oral Sex

In general, it may be possible to get some STIs in the mouth and throat from giving oral sex to a partner who is infected. This can include rectal infection and infection on the penis. It may also be possible to contract sexually transmitted infections (of the penis, vagina, anus, or rectum) by receiving oral sex from a partner who has an infection of the mouth or throat. It is possible to contract an STI transmitted through oral sex and for it spread to other parts of the body. Anilingus can transmit hepatitis A and B, intestinal parasites, and bacteria like E. coli.

Diseases that can be passed through oral sex include chlamydia, gonorrhea, syphilis, herpes, HPV, and HIV.

Having poor oral health, including tooth decay, gum disease, or oral cancer, can increase the chance of getting and transmitting disease. Also having open sores in the mouth and on the genitals can increase risk. Infection can also be passed through pre-ejaculatory fluids.

Risks of disease transmission through oral sex can be reduced by using a dental dam or a condom and reducing the number of sex partners.

Penile-Vaginal Intercourse

Many STIs are spread through contact with infected body fluids such as blood, vaginal fluids, or semen. Individuals of either sex can be exposed to infected body fluids and skin through penis-vagina sex.

Some sexually transmitted infections that can be passed this way include bacterial vaginosis, chancroid, gonorrhea, syphilis, hepatitis, herpes, HIV, HPV, crabs/pubic lice, pelvic inflammatory disease, trichomoniasis, and other less common infections.

Risk of STI transmission can be reduced by using condoms through the entire sex act (start to finish), reducing the number of sexual partners, using lubricants to reduce friction and tearing of condom or sensitive tissues, limiting or eliminating drug and alcohol use before sex, getting tested, having sexual partners get tested, and talking to health care providers about other prophylaxis methods if appropriate (PrEP or PEP for those at high risk of contracting HIV).

Anal Sex

Anal sex can be considered a high-risk sexual activity in terms of disease transmission for a couple different reasons. The lining of the anus is delicate and produces less natural lubricant than the vagina, which makes tissue tearing more likely. Additionally, due to fecal matter being present, tears are susceptible to infection and may be slower to heal. This makes contact with blood more likely, particularly if not using a condom.

Sexually transmitted infections can be transmitted both from giving and receiving anal sex, though transmission from receptive anal sex is most common. Some sexually transmitted infections that can be passed through anal sexual activity include chlamydia, chancroid, gonorrhea, granuloma inguinale, syphilis, hepatitis, herpes, HPV, and HIV.

Steps can be taken to make anal sex safer, including gently easing into anal sex and moving slowly, using plenty of lubrication, using a condom for the entire sexual experience (start to finish), avoiding spermicide which can irritate the rectum, never moving from anal sex to vaginal sex without first changing condom or washing, and stopping if there is severe pain during penetration.

Types of Sexually Transmitted Infections

Common sexually transmitted infections are generally classified as Nonviral/Bacterial STIs, Viral STIs, and Sexually Transmitted Parasitic Skin Infections. Many bacterial infections can be treated and cured with antibiotic medications. Some antibiotic-resistant strains have formed, however. Viral sexually transmitted infections are not treated with antibiotics, but some antiviral medications can be used for treatment. Most cannot be cured. Parasitic skin infections are typically treated using special shampoos and cream treatments. Some common sexually transmitted diseases are detailed below (summarized and adapted from information from the CDC).[45]

Bacterial Sexually Transmitted Infections

Bacterial Vaginosis (BV)—occurs when there is an overgrowth of a bacteria in the vagina, disrupting the normal bacterial balance. It is the most common vaginal condition in women ages fifteen to forty-four. The presence of BV can increase the risk of getting other sexually transmitted infections. Risk is increased through sexual contact, by having multiple sex partners, and by douching. Many do not experience symptoms, but if symptoms are present they may include thin white or gray vaginal discharge, pain or itching in the vagina, a strong fish-like odor particularly after sex, burning during urination, or itching around the vagina. A simple lab test of vaginal fluid is used to determine presence of BV. BV can be transmitted through female sex partners. Untreated BV can increase risk of contracting chlamydia, gonorrhea, and other STIs. It can sometimes cause pelvic inflammatory disease which can limit fertility.

Gonorrhea—can infect the cervix, urethra, rectum, or throat. It is very common and particularly prevalent in people ages fifteen to twenty-four. It can be passed through sexual contact or by pregnant women to their children during childbirth. Symptoms can be mild or absent in women and men. If symptoms are present in men, they may include burning during urination, white, yellow, or green discharge from the penis, or painful or swollen testicles. Women may experience pain or burning during urination, increased vaginal discharge, or bleeding between periods. Rectal infections can be asymptomatic or include anal discharge, itching, soreness, bleeding, or painful bowel movements. Sexually active people can reduce risk by limiting sex partners, getting tested, encouraging partners to get tested, and using latex condoms correctly every time a person has sex. Usually a urine test is used to detect gonorrhea. If an individual had oral or anal sex, it is important to collect samples from the throat and/or rectum. Sometimes a sample is taken from the male's urethra or a woman's cervix. Gonorrhea can typically be cured with antibiotics, although drug-resistant strains are increasing. If left untreated, gonorrhea can cause serious health problems for men and women, including pelvic inflammatory disease in women (limiting fertility), increasing the risk of ectopic pregnancy, infertility, and long-term pelvic/abdominal pain. In men, untreated gonorrhea can cause a painful condition that can limit fertility. It can (rarely) spread to blood and joints, creating life-threatening complications. Delaying treatment can also increase the risks of contracting HIV.

Syphilis—can cause serious health problems if left untreated. Without treatment, it progresses through stages (primary, secondary, latent, and tertiary). Each stage has unique symptoms. Primary syphilis is characterized by the presence of a sore (or sores) at the site of infection. The sores are usually firm, round, and painless. With progression to secondary syphilis, the individual develops a rash, swollen lymph nodes, and a fever. The symptoms may be mild and unnoticed. In the latent stage, there are no symptoms. With progression to the tertiary stage, the individual will experience serious medical problems including complications in the heart, brain, and other organs. Risk of syphilis can be reduced by limiting sex partners, being tested, only having sexual contact with a partner who has been tested, and correctly using latex condoms from start to finish. Usually a blood sample or fluid from a sore is used to test for syphilis. Syphilis can be treated with antibiotics, but damage caused by the infection cannot be undone.

Chlamydia—is a common STI that can impact fertility and increase the risk of fatal ectopic pregnancy if not treated. Many who are infected do not show symptoms. If present, symptoms include genital discharge and burning during urination. Women may experience pain in lower abdomen or pain during intercourse, but in most cases women have no symptoms. People can reduce their risk of acquiring chlamydia if sexually active by limiting the number of sexual partners and using condoms correctly during intercourse. Sexually active young people are at greater risk of getting chlamydia. Sexually active women younger than age twenty-five should be tested every year. Lab tests with urine or vaginal swabs can determine if someone has chlamydia. It can usually be cured with antibiotic treatment.

Trichomoniasis—is a common sexually transmitted disease caused by an infection with a parasite. In women, the most common infection site is the lower genital tract including the vulva, vagina, cervix, or urethra. In men, the most common site is the urethra. It can spread from the vagina to the penis, the penis to the vagina, or from the vagina to another vagina. It can also infect the hands, mouth, or anus. Most people will not show symptoms if infected, but if they do, men may notice itching inside the penis, burning after urination or ejaculation, or discharge from the penis; women may notice itching, burning, redness or soreness of the genitals, discomfort with urination, a change in vaginal discharge that can be clear, white, yellowish, or greenish with a fishy smell. Untreated trichomoniasis can increase the risk of getting or spreading other STIs and can increase the risk of preterm delivery and low-birthweight birth in women who are pregnant. Lab tests are used to diagnose trichomoniasis. Oral medications are used to treat the disease. Risk of transmission can be reduced in those sexually active by limiting the number of sex partners, getting tested, encouraging partners to get tested, and using latex condoms correctly every time you have sex.

Viral Sexually Transmitted Infections

Herpes—is an STI that is caused by two types of viruses—herpes simplex type 1 (HSV-1) and herpes simplex type 2 (HSV-2). Although sometimes distinguished as "oral herpes" and "genital herpes," infection of both types can occur in the genitals. Oral herpes is usually caused by HSV-1, causing cold sores around the mouth. Most people with HSV-1 will not show symptoms. It can be passed by nonsexual contact. Oral herpes can also be transmitted to the genitals through oral sex. Genital herpes is very common and is spread through contact with a herpes sore, contact with saliva (if a partner is infected with oral herpes) and genital secretions (if a partner is infected with HSV-2), and contact with skin of person who is infected (oral area or genital area). Transmission can occur when no symptoms are present, but likelihood of transmission is increased during active outbreaks. Risk can be reduced by limiting the number of sexual partners and using latex condoms and dental dams correctly every time you have vaginal, anal, or oral sex. If engaging in sexual activity with someone who is infected, make sure they take their medication every day and avoid having vaginal, anal, or oral sex when an infected partner demonstrates symptoms.

The first outbreak of HSV-2 is typically the most severe. It may include painful blisters around the genitals and rectum. Individuals may also experience flu-like symptoms including fever, body aches, or swollen glands. Repeated outbreaks can occur. The infection stays in the body for the rest of the person's life and the symptoms may lessen over time. To test for genital herpes, the doctor will likely just look at symptoms or they may take a sample from a sore if sores are present. Sometimes a blood test is used to check for antibodies. Herpes can also be passed to other areas by touching sores and then touching other parts of the body. Herpes, particularly during active outbreaks with open sores, can increase risk of acquiring other STIs.

Although there is no cure, medications can reduce the number of outbreaks and can reduce the risk of transmitting it to others.

Human Papillomavirus (HPV)—is the most commonly transmitted STI and consists of many types of viruses. Some of the types cause genital warts and some types cause cancers. It is most commonly spread through vaginal and anal sex. Many people who are infected show no symptoms, or it can be years before symptoms are present. Most of the time, the body clears it on its own and it doesn't cause any negative consequences. Genital warts can appear as a small bump or as a group of bumps around the genitals and anus. Cancer causing strains of HPV can cause cancers of the uterine cervix, vulva, penis, anus, throat, tongue, and tonsils. Risk of transmission can be decreased by getting screened for cervical cancer (recommended routinely for women ages twenty-one to sixty-five), getting vaccinated, using latex condoms and dental dams correctly every time you have sex, reducing the number of sex partners, and being in a mutually monogamous relationship. Vaccination is recommended at age eleven or twelve and for everyone through age twenty-six. Some adults ages twenty-seven to forty-five may also choose to get vaccinated. There is no test to assess HPV status, but tests can be used to assess cervical cancer status. Genital warts can be treated with medication or simply left alone. Cervical precancer can be treated with a variety of medical treatments. HPV cancers are more treatable if caught early with rapid treatment.

Hepatitis A and B—are diseases impacting the liver, causing inflammation and impacting function. Hepatitis A is spread sexually through fecal-oral contact and typically doesn't show symptoms right away, but can cause fatigue, nausea, vomiting, abdominal pain, clay-colored bowel movements, loss of appetite, low-grade fever, dark urine, yellowing of the skin, itching, and joint pain several weeks after exposure. Getting a vaccine for hepatitis A can reduce the risk of becoming infected. Transmission is more common in MSM and in those who are HIV positive. Type A does not cause long-term liver damage or become chronic. Reducing sexual transmission can be assisted by abstaining from oral contact with the anus, reducing the number of sexual partners, and using latex condoms and dental dams (particularly when performing anilingus).

Hepatitis B can become chronic and can increase the risk of developing liver failure, liver cancer, and liver cirrhosis. A vaccine can also prevent hepatitis B. Symptoms are similar to hepatitis A. When Hepatitis B is spread through sexual contact, it is passed through contact with blood, saliva, semen, or vaginal secretions. With acute infection, hepatitis B clears from the body and recovery occurs in a matter of months. With chronic infection, hepatitis B lasts six months or more and may even last a lifetime. People can avoid sexual transmission of HBV by knowing the status of those with whom they have sexual contact, reducing the number of sex partners, using condoms correctly every time, and avoiding illicit drugs.

Acquired Immunodeficiency Syndrome (AIDS)—is a chronic condition caused by the HIV virus. HIV interferes with the body's ability to fight infection. HIV is transmitted sexually by contact with blood, semen, or vaginal secretions. Some people develop a flu-like illness within weeks of the virus entering the body. In the clinical latent infection stage, HIV is still present in the body and in white blood cells, but people may not have symptoms. This stage can last for many years. As it progresses to symptomatic HIV infection, if untreated, it will multiply and destroy immune cells and the individual may develop infections and chronic signs and symptoms. If the infection is untreated and progresses to AIDS, the immune system is severely damaged. Individuals in this stage are more likely to develop opportunistic infection or cancers. Risk of transmission can be reduced by limiting sex partners, getting male circumcision, treating other STIs, abstaining from IV drug use, and using condoms correctly every time. The use of pre-exposure prophylaxis (PrEP) (antiviral medications used to prevent HIV negative persons from becoming positive) can reduce the risk of sexually transmitted HIV in very high-risk groups. The use of post-exposure prophylaxis (PEP) (emergency medications that are used if one suspects they have been exposure to HIV through sexual contact or through sharing needles) can reduce risk if taken within seventy-two hours of possible exposure. Treatment with medication among those who are positive can reduce viral load and reduce the risk of transmitting infection to others.

Sexually Transmitted Parasitic Skin Infections

Pubic lice (crabs)—are parasites that feed on the skin in the pubic area, causing blue and gray spots. They are typically spread through sexual contact. The lice and their eggs (nits) are tiny but can be seen with the human eye. Lice can live for a short time on towels, clothing, and bedding. Pubic lice feed on blood and can cause severe itching. Treatment includes the use of a special shampoo or lotion that kills their eggs. Hair removal alone is not likely sufficient.

Scabies—is an itchy skin condition caused by a burrowing, female mite. Intense itching occurs at the burrow site and irregular burrow tracks of tiny blisters may appear. Scabies is contagious through close physical contact. Burrowing is likely to appear between the fingers, in the armpits, around the waist, along the inside of wrists, on the inner elbows, on the soles of the feet, around the breasts, around the male genitalia, on the buttocks, and on the knees. If diagnosed, most physicians will recommend treatment for all in the home or contact group. Transmission occurs when the mite burrows beneath the skin and deposits eggs; they hatch, and they work their way to the surface where they spread to other parts of the body or to other people. Scabies can spread when people share bedding or clothing. Risk can be reduced by cleaning all clothes and linens and sealing infected garments for a couple of weeks to kill any living mites.

CHAPTER NINE

....

Birth Control

How Do All These Things Work Anyway?

For better or for worse, like it or not, the risk of pregnancy is usually present in heterosexual intercourse among individuals who are of childbearing age and ability. So for most people engaging in heterosexual sex (including, unfortunately, nonconsensual sex), there will always be some level of risk. At the same time, there have never been more options for birth control available for most who choose to be sexually active. Regardless of this broad theoretical access, according to the Centers for Disease Control and Prevention (CDC), about 50 percent of pregnancies in the US are unintended.[46] And among teens ages fifteen to nineteen, that number climbs to 75 percent. In the US, some factors that increase the risk of unintended pregnancy include being eighteen to twenty-four years old, having low income (less than 100 percent of Federal Poverty Level), not completing high school, being a non-Hispanic Black or of African American ethnicity, and cohabitating without marriage. Additionally, a multitude of factors can limit an individual's ability to access birth control. Some of these factors include cost, geographical access issues, religious/ethical/moral/political objections, health limitations, embarrassment, lack of knowledge, lack of empowerment, and lack of health insurance.

Successfully avoiding pregnancy, if that is the desired outcome, requires effectively reaching several goals. Both partners must first accept and understand that sexual activity places them at risk of pregnancy. (You wouldn't believe how many students have said things to me like, "I heard that if you douche with soda after sex you can't get pregnant," or, "I heard that if you jump up and down after sex you cannot get pregnant," or, "I heard you can't get pregnant if it is your first time.") The person or partners must then obtain appropriate and accurate information about birth control methods and based on that decide which to use. (There is an inordinate amount of false information that travels among friends and on the internet about birth control methods.) And then the individual or individuals must use the method properly and consistently. There are many things that can get in the way of reaching those three goals. Effective education, planning, and open communication can improve the likelihood of achieving each.

Statistically, the desired family size in the US is two children. According to the Guttmacher Institute, to achieve that goal, a heterosexual woman would need to use contraceptives for about three decades. Although many parents wish for their children to remain sexually abstinent, most people will eventually become sexually active and wish to use some form of birth control at some point. Additionally, many young people engage in sexual behavior and may benefit from fact-based information that they are statistically unlikely to get at school or from other credible sources. Age-appropriate, honest discussions about birth control can have many benefits and empower people to make informed decisions about their health and safety.

The question that I am undoubtedly asked most when speaking to people about birth control options is "Yeah...but...which type is best?" Choosing birth control is more complex than just deciding which is "best." Many individual factors must be considered when choosing between birth control options. Understanding the types that are available, levels of individual comfort, risks involved with use, level of personal accountability involved in use, theoretical and practical efficacy, cost, and other considerations can make for a more appropriate and informed decision. It is also important to note that birth control preferences may change with age and life situations. Teens and younger women may prefer long-acting but reversible methods like IUDs and implants that don't require them to think about birth control on a daily basis like they would with birth control pills. Individuals in committed, monogamous relationships may make different birth control choices than those in different types of relationships. People who engage in sexual intercourse infrequently may be less likely to want to use hormonal methods and may prefer to use a barrier method. Later in life or, if choosing not to have children, some may be more interested in permanent methods of birth control. For these reasons and others, it makes sense to regularly assess which methods are most appropriate given current lifestyle-related factors.

Some questions that may be important to consider when exploring options for birth control include:

- What level of protection is needed?

- How often am I engaging in sexual contact?

- Do I need a method that prevents both pregnancy and sexually transmitted infection?

- Am I or is my partner comfortable inserting a device into the vaginal canal?

- Am I comfortable with my ability to remember to think about birth control daily? Or do I trust my partner to remember it daily?

- Am I comfortable with my ability to remember to use birth control during the "heat of the moment?"

- Do I have moral or religious objections to certain methods of birth control?

- What is my budget for birth control? What can I or my partner afford?

- Do I have health insurance or other access to birth control? What types of birth control methods are covered? Are there copays involved? How much of a supply can I get per visit?

- Do I have any relevant allergies or health conditions that exclude certain options?

- Do I or my partner want to become pregnant soon? What are my goals for my future?

- Am I willing or able to obtain a doctor's visit to get access to birth control?

- Have I discussed concerns, hesitations, and preferences regarding birth control methods with my partner?

- Am I a smoker?

- Am I overweight or obese?

- Have I given birth before or had an abortion?

Many types of birth control are described below including comments regarding their safety, efficacy, how they work, how long they last, how they are obtained, pros and cons regarding use, and special considerations. *The following descriptions of birth control methods are meant to be summaries and are not inclusive of all individual risk and benefits. The summaries are not designed to be comprehensive descriptions or to replace medical advice.*[47]

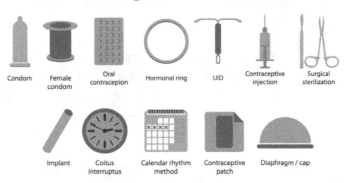

Contraception methods

Condom   Female condom   Oral contracepion   Hormonal ring   UID   Contraceptive injection   Surgical sterilization

Implant   Coitus interruptus   Calendar rhythm method   Contraceptive patch   Diaphragm / cap

Hormonal Methods of Birth Control

There are many types of birth control that use hormones to prevent pregnancy. Many work in similar ways and have similar benefits and risks depending on the types of hormones they contain and personal characteristics of the user. Some brand names are listed below, and many also have generic forms available.

Birth Control Pill (Combination)

Combination birth control pills are oral contraceptives that contain a type of estrogen and progestin. There are a variety of types of combination birth control pills. They prevent pregnancy by preventing ovulation (the release of the egg from the ovary), thinning the lining of the uterus, and thickening the mucus on the cervix, which serves as somewhat of a "plug" which makes it more difficult for sperm to enter into the uterus.

Additionally, combination pills come in both continuous-dosing or conventional-dosing form.

Conventional-dosing packs usually contain twenty-one "active" pills and seven "inactive" pills, or twenty-four active pills and four inactive pills. The active pills contain hormones and the inactive pills do not. A person taking conventional packs will generally experience bleeding every month while taking the inactive pills.

Continuous-dosing or extended-cycle packs usually contain eighty-four active pills and seven inactive pills. Bleeding typically occurs while taking the inactive pills. Some packs contain only active pills which eliminates bleeding altogether.

Some combination pill packs contain equal amounts of estrogen and progestin in each active pill (monophasic) and others have varying amounts (multiphasic).

Some find that combination birth control pills help relieve PMS symptoms and decrease the severity of menstrual cramps, decrease blood flow during periods, reduce acne, and create more predictable periods. Benefits also may include a reduction in risk of endometriosis, and a decreased risk of ovarian, endometrial, and colorectal cancers. Some people who are not sexually active choose to take combination birth control due to these benefits.

Combination pills must be taken at the same time every day in order to be most effective, which can be a barrier for some. (There are apps that can help with this and some may find it helpful to just set a daily reminder alarm to assist.) Combination pills provide no protection against sexually transmitted infections. They may cause irregular bleeding, bloating, breast tenderness, nausea, depression, weight gain, and headache in some.

They also may increase the risk of blood clots, especially for smokers and women who are over the age of thirty-five. They may increase the risk of high cholesterol, heart attack, and stroke. They require a prescription by a doctor, and if someone chooses to use combination birth control pills, they can work with their health care providers to determine which type is most appropriate. There are many types available that contain varying levels of hormones, so if one type is not tolerated well, there are possibly other options that may work better. Fertility is likely to resume quickly after cessation.

Birth Control Pill (Progestin-Only or "Mini-Pill")

The progestin-only pill, also called the mini-pill, is an oral contraceptive that prevents pregnancy by thickening the cervical mucus so that sperm cannot reach the egg, and by thinning the lining of the uterus. It may also prevent ovulation but does not do so consistently. The mini-pill does not contain estrogen, so it is safe to use while breastfeeding. Others may choose to use the mini-pill if they have a history of blood clots in the legs or lungs or if they are concerned about side effects from estrogen. Fertility is likely to resume quickly after cessation.

Unlike the combination pill, the progestin-only pill packs do not contain inactive pills. The progestin-only pill has a higher failure rate than the combination pill and about thirteen out of a hundred women who use it will get pregnant in a year of use. It is very important that the mini-pill be taken at the same time every day, a routine some find difficult to strictly adhere to. If the pill is taken more than three hours late, it is necessary to plan on a backup method or abstinence to avoid pregnancy. Side effects may include irregular menstrual bleeding, acne, breast tenderness, decreased sex drive, depression, headaches, nausea, ovarian cysts, and even increased risk of ectopic pregnancy if pregnancy does occur. The pill does not provide any protection against STIs. A doctor visit and prescription are necessary to obtain the progestin-only pill.

Birth Control Patch

The birth control patch is hormonal birth control that contains estrogen and progestin. The patch works similarly to oral combination pills. It prevents pregnancy by preventing ovulation (the release of the egg from the ovary), thinning the lining of the uterus, and thickening the mucus on the cervix.

The patch is placed on the skin once a week for three weeks and left off the fourth week; when it is left off, menstrual bleeding occurs. It can be placed on the lower abdomen, buttocks, or upper body (but not on the breasts). The patch requires a prescription from a health care provider and does not protect against STIs.

Some women like that the patch does not require them to think about contraception every day or with each sexual act. It also allows a woman to take control of her own fertility without requiring a partner's cooperation. Side effects may include spotting, skin irritation, breast tenderness and pain, menstrual pain, headaches, nausea and vomiting, abdominal pain, and an increased risk of blood-clotting problems, heart attack, stroke, liver cancer, gallbladder disease and high blood pressure, vaginal infections, fluid retention, weight gain, mood swings, and acne. According to a statement from the Mayo Clinic, "Research shows that the birth control patch may increase estrogen levels in the body compared to combination birth control pills that are taken by mouth. You may have a slightly higher risk of estrogen-related adverse events, such as blood clots, while using the patch than if you took combination birth control pills."[48]

Health care providers may advise against its use if an individual has a history of heart attack, stroke, severe high blood pressure, or they are over thirty-five and smoke. They may also discourage use if there is a history of breast, uterine, or liver cancer or if the individual weighs more than 198 pounds. Some with skin sensitivities, certain medication use, or other conditions may also be advised against use.

The patch is very effective, and less than one out of a hundred women will get pregnant during the first year of typical use of the birth control patch.

Birth Control Implant (Brand Name Nexplanon)

The contraceptive implant is a long-term birth control method that works by releasing a steady dose of a progestational hormone into the bloodstream. A health care provider places the flexible, plastic, matchstick shaped rod under the skin of the upper arm. The implant works by thickening cervical mucus and the lining of the uterus; it also typically suppresses ovulation.

Some prefer this hormonal method because it does not contain estrogen, does not require the individual to think about birth control often, and can be removed at any time with restored fertility. It can be left in for several years and less than one pregnancy per one hundred women will occur for one year of use. It is removed by a trained health care provider in a minor surgical procedure.

Women using the implant may notice changes to their normal menstrual bleeding or have no bleeding at all. The implant may increase the risk of blood clots, especially in women with risk factors like smoking. Additionally, according to the Nexplanon website, "other common side effects reported in women using Nexplanon include: headaches; vaginitis (inflammation of the vagina); weight gain; acne; breast pain; viral infection such as sore throats or flu-like symptoms; stomach pain; painful periods; mood swings, nervousness, or depressed mood; back pain; nausea; dizziness; pain and pain at the site of insertion. Implants have been reported to be found in a blood vessel, including a blood vessel in the lung."[49] Other individual preexisting conditions may also make an implant an inappropriate option for birth control. Consulting with a health care provider is a great way to determine if the implant is a good option. It does not protect against STIs.

Intrauterine Device (IUD) (Brand Names Paragard, Mirena, Kyleena, Liletta, and Skyla)

An IUD is a small flexible plastic device that is shaped like a *T* and placed by a health care provide into the uterus. At the time of this publication, there are five different brands of IUDs that are FDA approved for use in the United States, including Paragard, Mirena, Kyleena, Liletta, and Skyla. IUDs come in two types that work differently. One is considered a copper type (Paragard) and the others are considered hormonal types (Mirena, Kyleena, Liletta, and Skyla).

Copper IUDs protect individuals from pregnancy for up to twelve years. They work by changing the way sperm cells move in order to prevent them from reaching the egg. Some also use the copper IUD as emergency contraception. If placed within 120 hours (five days) following unprotected sex, it is more than 99.9 percent effective at preventing pregnancy.

Hormonal IUDs work in two different ways. They thicken cervical mucus and sometimes prevent ovulation. Hormonal IUDs are left in up to three to seven years depending on type.

Both can be removed at any time and fertility restored. Because they do not contain estrogen, they can safely be used by people who are breastfeeding.

Many enjoy IUDs because they provide long-lasting protection that involves very little risk of human error or effort on the part of the user. Once they are placed, the user can pretty much forget about them.

Potential side effects include pain upon placement, cramping following placement, spotting and irregular periods, and heavier periods with copper IUDs.

During placement, a health care provider will insert a speculum and then use an inserter to place the IUD through the opening of the cervix and into the uterus. They may first offer medication that helps to open and numb the cervix. People generally report some cramping or pain with placement. Some will experience cramping and spotting for several months after insertion. Some people will then experience lighter periods or no period at all. With copper IUDs, some report heavier periods with more cramping. Copper IUDs begin preventing pregnancy as soon as they are placed, and hormonal IUDs may require a backup method for a specified time depending on timing of placement.

IUDs may not be appropriate for people with certain STDs or current or recent pelvic infections. They may not be a good option for people who think they may be pregnant, have untreated cervical cancer or cancer of breast or the uterus. Bleeding disorders, allergies, or uterus shape may limit options or make IUDs an inappropriate birth control option.

IUDs are one of the most effective types of birth control, with fewer than one out of a hundred people becoming pregnant with IUD use each year.

Birth Control Shot (Brand Name Depo Provera)

The birth control shot is an injection that is given in the arm or buttocks every three months to prevent pregnancy. The shot contains progestin that works to thicken cervical mucus and helps to prevent ovulation. The most commonly used birth control shot is brand name Depo Provera.

Some individuals prefer this method because it is private and only needs to be thought about four times a year. Most women using this method have lighter periods or no periods at all.

Disadvantages include no protection against STIs and a required visit to the health care provider every twelve weeks; for some it may take longer to become pregnant (possibly ten months or more) after cessation, and continued use (two or more years) may cause a reduction in bone mineral density that is possibly irreversible. The FDA recommends that individuals not take Depo Provera longer than two years and warns that use may increase the risk of osteoporosis and bone fractures later in life. Other side effects may include breast tenderness, spotting, weight gain, depression, dizziness, nervousness, abdominal discomfort, and headaches. People who are averse to needles may not want to get an injection every twelve weeks. Additionally, for some it may take five or more months for fertility to return after discontinuing injections, though there is certainly no guarantee of that. The birth control shot is probably not ideal for people wishing to get pregnant right away after stopping use.

Vaginal Ring (Brand Names NuvaRing and Annovera)

The vaginal ring is hormonal birth control made from flexible, latex-free plastic that is inserted into the vaginal canal. It contains both estrogen and progestin which are slowly released over a three-week period. After three weeks, the ring is removed for a week which allows menstrual bleeding to occur. Some may choose to insert another ring directly after removal to avoid menstruation.

The ring prevents pregnancy by preventing ovulation, thickening cervical mucus, and thinning the lining of the uterus. At the time of this publication, two vaginal ring hormonal contraceptive devices are approved by the FDA including the NuvaRing and Annovera. Both require a prescription from a health care provider.

Some may choose this option because vaginal rings are easy to use and don't require thinking about birth control every day or with each sexual encounter. Women don't have to be individually fitted for use and vaginal rings can be inserted and removed at home by the user. They also deliver a relatively small amount of hormones throughout the body which some may find desirable. They can be removed at any time and allow for quick return to fertility. They are less likely to cause irregular bleeding or weight gain than some other hormonal birth control methods.

Vaginal rings require that the individual be comfortable performing its proper insertion and removal, so may not be the best option for people who are uncomfortable reaching into the vaginal canal. They may not be appropriate for people older than thirty-five or those who smoke. They may also be inappropriate for people with diabetes or blood-vessel complications including blood clots, history of breast, uterine, or liver cancer or disease. They may not be recommended for people with migraines, high blood pressure, unexplained vaginal bleeding or other conditions or medication use.

Emergency Contraception (for Use after Unprotected Sex Has Occurred)

"Morning-After Pills"

Levonorgestrel emergency contraceptive (brand name Plan B, generics and other brands) is used after unprotected sex or failure of other forms of birth control (i.e., broken condom, missing birth control pills, etc.). It is a progestin-only contraception that works by delaying or stopping ovulation and interfering with fertilization and potentially altering the lining of the uterus, similar to the way a birth control pill works. It contains the same hormone that is in regular birth control pills at a higher dose. It is a single pill that is taken as soon as possible after unprotected sex within seventy-two hours. It is not meant to be used as a regular birth control method and will not protect against STIs. Plan B is not recommended for women who weigh more than 165 pounds or whose body mass index (BMI) is above 25 kg/m^2.

Although many misconceptions exist, because it works by preventing ovulation, this type of emergency contraception will help prevent pregnancy before it starts but will not affect an existing pregnancy. It is not the same as RU-486 and does not cause miscarriage or abortion. It will not stop the development of a fetus once implantation into the uterus has occurred.

The sooner the emergency contraception pill is taken the more effective it is. If taken within twenty-four hours of unprotected sex, it is about 95 percent effective at preventing pregnancy. If taken within seventy-two hours of unprotected sex, it can reduce the risk of pregnancy by about 89 percent. Depending on where a person lives, it can be purchased over the counter without a prescription at drug stores and other locations and in some places even in vending machines.

Like with other types of hormonal contraception, some side effects may include changes in menstrual period (lighter, heavier, earlier, late), nausea, lower-abdominal cramps, tiredness, headache, dizziness, breast tenderness, and vomiting.

Ulipristal Acetate Tablet (brand name Ella and generics) or the morning-after pill (brand name Ella) is a single pill containing an active ingredient called ulipristal acetate; it is given by prescription and works by delaying or preventing ovulation. It may also make it difficult for the egg to imbed into the uterus if it has been fertilized. It is more effective than progestin-only emergency contraception and it can be used later than Plan B following unprotected sex (up to five days vs. three with progestin-only emergency contraception). It can be ordered online and, in some states, a pharmacist can provide a prescription. It can also be obtained at family planning clinics, campus/student health centers, urgent care and emergency rooms or from healthcare providers. It lowers a person's chance of getting pregnant by 85 percent if taken within five days (120 hours) of having unprotected sex. Ella and other forms of emergency contraceptives may be less effective in women with a BMI above 30 kg/m^2. Ella has less stringent weight requirements than with Plan B and may be effective for larger women. If vomiting within three hours of taking the pill occurs, it may be less likely to work.

As with other forms of hormonal contraception, some side effects may include headache, nausea, stomach pain, menstrual pain or cramps, tiredness, or dizziness.

Copper IUD (Brand Name Paragard)

Can be used as contraception or emergency contraception. See section above for details.

Medication Abortion (Brand Name Mifepristone and Misoprostol, Mifegymiso)

Mifepristone and misoprostol (Mifegymiso, the combination of the two) are used to chemically induce abortion and are given by prescription. The medication mifepristone is a synthetic steroid that works to terminate intrauterine pregnancy by blocking the body's own progesterone, which inhibits the maturation of a pregnancy. When mifepristone is followed by misoprostol (either right away or up to forty-eight hours later), cramping of the uterus is induced to induce the shedding and emptying of the uterus. This will resemble a heavy, cramping period or early miscarriage.

If used within eight weeks or less of pregnancy, it is about 94 to 98 percent effective. For people who are ten to eleven weeks pregnant, it is about 87 percent effective. Extra dosage can enhance efficacy. In general, individuals can be prescribed medication abortion up to eleven weeks after the first day of the last period.

Some possible side effects include bleeding, cramping, pelvic pain, nausea, diarrhea, stomach pain, dizziness, tiredness, weakness, back pain, and allergic reaction such as closing of the throat, swelling of the lips, tongue, or face. Medication may also interact with other prescriptions. Follow-up medical appointments are also recommended after using mifepristone and misoprostol.

Although these medicines are available online, it should be noted that many dangerous, nonapproved, and ineffective medications are sold over the internet. Consumers should use caution, particularly with abortion-inducing medications.

Barrier Methods

(External) Condom

External condoms, sometimes called male condoms or just condoms, are thin pouches made of latex, plastics, or lambskin that cover the penis during vaginal, oral, or anal sex. Condoms are effective at reducing the spread of sexually transmitted infections and preventing pregnancy if used correctly. Condoms made of lambskin or other animal membranes are not effective for preventing transmission of STIs, including HIV.

External condoms prevent pregnancy by creating a barrier between semen and the uterine cervix, preventing fertilization from occurring. With perfect use they are about 98 percent effective at preventing pregnancy. But typical use is closer to about 85 percent, so learning how to use condoms effectively is a very important component of sexual empowerment!

A person can increase the efficacy of condoms for contraception by using them correctly every time, using them in conjunction with another method of birth control (like the pill), or adding spermicide. Only one condom should be used at a time (no doubling up).

Many enjoy condoms as a form of birth control because they are inexpensive (and often can be obtained for free in family planning clinics and other places), help to protect against the spread of STIs, and do not require ingesting hormones. Disadvantages may include that they require proper use during the "heat of the moment," need to be readily available every time, may change sensation of sexual intercourse, and are not a female-controlled method.

Read more about using external condoms in Chapter Seven.

(Internal) Condom

Like external condoms, internal condoms (sometimes called female condoms) are inserted into the vaginal canal (or can be inserted into the anus) to prevent pregnancy by blocking sperm from entering the cervix; they also provide protection against the spread of STIs. They are made from a soft plastic that looks like a pouch with a ring at the end and the base. The inner ring is squeezed and inserted into the vaginal canal and then attaches to the cervix. The external ring wraps around the vulva on the outside of the body covering some of the vulva. They are more expensive than external condoms, are less available, and are less effective with typical use. With perfect use they are about 95 percent effective. But typical use is closer to about 79 percent effective. Some women prefer them because they allow them to be in control of their use. Some prefer the feel of them because they don't fit tightly around the penis. Some enjoy the way that the inner ring feels on the penis. Some women enjoy the way that the external ring may rub against the vulva and clitoris. They are also latex-free which may be desirable for those with sensitive skin.

Effectiveness can be enhanced by wearing them for the entire sexual experience and using them every single time a person has vaginal sex (also using them every time an individual has anal sex for STI protection). Efficacy is also improved by combining it with other contraceptive methods (like the pill or an IUD). DO NOT use them in conjunction with another external (male) condom.

Diaphragm

The diaphragm provides contraception by creating a barrier between the cervix and semen. It is made from soft silicone and is shaped like a small saucer. It is inserted with spermicide before intercourse by bending it in half and sliding it into the vaginal canal until it reaches the cervix where it expands. It can be placed up to two hours before having intercourse and needs to be left in at least six hours after the last time the person has sex and for no more than twenty-four hours. When used perfectly each time, it is about 94 percent effective at preventing pregnancy. With typical use, it is closer to 88 percent effective. Efficacy can be improved by using it for every sexual encounter, using it with spermicide every time, ensuring that it is covering the cervix, using it with another form of birth control like condoms, and having sexual partners pull out before ejaculating. Diaphragms alone do not provide protection against STIs.

An individual needs to be fitted for their diaphragm by a medical provider. After receiving a prescription, it can be purchased at a pharmacy, drugstore, or health center. It works best for people who are comfortable placing and removing it, are not allergic to silicone or spermicide, haven't recently given birth, haven't had toxic shock syndrome, and haven't had an abortion in the second or third trimester within the last six weeks.

Side effects may include urinary tract infections (UTIs) and vaginal irritation and other side effects associated with spermicide use.

Weight fluctuation may change the efficacy of the diaphragm. Individuals should get refitted if losing or gaining ten or more pounds.

Birth Control Sponge (Brand Name Today Sponge)

Like the diaphragm, the birth control sponge provides contraception by creating a barrier between the cervix and semen. It is made from soft, spongy plastic. It contains spermicide and is inserted before intercourse into the vaginal canal until it reaches the cervix. Before insertion, the sponge should be wetted with clean water and squeezed until sudsy. It has a fabric loop on it which can be pulled on to remove it. The sponge is most effective when used by women who have not given birth. When used perfectly by women who are nulliparous, it is about 91 percent effective with perfect use. With typical use in that population, it is about 88 percent effective. Among those who have given birth, perfect use is about 80 percent, typical use 76 percent. Combing the sponge with another form of birth control, like the condom, will increase effectiveness. Having the partner "pull out" before ejaculating will also reduce the risk of pregnancy. By itself, the sponge does not provide protection against STIs.

It can be placed up to twenty-four hours before having intercourse and needs to be left in at least six hours after the last time the person has sex and for no more than thirty hours total.

The only approved sponge brand available in the US is the Today Sponge. It is available without a prescription and without age restriction from drugstores, pharmacies, family planning clinics, and some grocery stores.

The sponge may not be recommended for people who are allergic to spermicides, sulfites, or polyurethane. It also may be inappropriate for those who are not comfortable with placing or removing it, who have recently had a birth, abortion or miscarriage, who have a vaginal infection or history of toxic shock syndrome; or who are currently menstruating.

Side effects may include UTIs and vaginal irritation and other side effects associated with spermicide use as well as a slightly increased risk of toxic shock syndrome. Nonoxynol-9, a spermicide used in the sponge, can also irritate the skin and possibly increase the risk of acquiring HIV and other STIs if exposed.

Some prefer to use a sponge for contraception because it doesn't require hormone use, can be used while breastfeeding, doesn't interrupt sex (allowing for spontaneity), and leaves the female in control.

Cervical Cap (Brand Name FemCap)

This cervical cap is made from soft silicone and covers the uterine cervix, creating a barrier between the cervix and semen in order to prevent pregnancy. Like the diaphragm and the sponge, it is used with spermicide. It is smaller than a diaphragm and slightly different in shape (more like a hat than a dish). The cervical cap can be left in up to two days (which is longer than the diaphragm and sponge). However, the diaphragm is more effective at preventing pregnancy. The cervical cap is more effective when used by those who have never given birth, and in that population is about 86 percent effective at preventing pregnancy. Among those who have given birth, efficacy is at about 71 percent.

Effectiveness can be enhanced by combining it with other methods (like condom use), pulling out before ejaculation, and using it correctly every time an individual has sex. Like the other internal barrier methods, it needs to be left for at least six hours after the last time the individual has sex and for no more than forty-eight hours. Used alone it does not provide protection against STIs.

Cervical caps are available with a prescription from a pharmacy, drugstore, family planning clinic, or health care center. They come in three different sizes. The appropriate size is determined by the health care provider.

The cervical cap may not be appropriate for those who are not comfortable with its insertion or removal, who have given birth or have had an abortion within the last six weeks, have allergies to silicone or spermicide, have cancer or other conditions of the cervix, are positive for HIV or have a partner who is, or have had toxic shock syndrome. Nonoxynol-9, a spermicide used with the cap, can also irritate the skin and possibly increase risk of acquiring HIV and other STIs if exposed. Cervical caps can also lose efficacy with weight gain. A person should be refitted with weight change and after having a baby, miscarriage, or abortion.

Some prefer to use a cap for contraception because it doesn't require hormone use, can be used while breastfeeding, doesn't interrupt sex (allowing for spontaneity), and leaves the female in control. Additionally, cervical caps, unlike sponges, can be used for a year with appropriate care.

Fertility Awareness Methods

Fertility awareness methods, sometimes referred to as "natural family planning" or the "rhythm method," work by tracking ovulation in order to predict fertile periods. They are used by some to increase the chance of getting pregnant and by others to determine which days to avoid intercourse in order to prevent pregnancy. Three methods that can assist in predicting ovulation include: the temperature method, the cervical mucus method, and the calendar method. Some use these methods in isolation or any or all of them in combination. There are also apps that can assist with tracking these metrics. Some women also rely on exclusive breastfeeding to reduce risk of pregnancy following childbirth, called the lactational amenorrhea method.

There are many reasons some may use fertility awareness methods, including religious and moral practice. Fertility awareness methods are about 76 to 88 percent effective, meaning that twelve to twenty-four out of a hundred couples who use this method as a form of birth control will get pregnant if used for a year. These methods are more effective when used together. They are less effective for those with irregular menstrual cycles, those who struggle to avoid sex during risky days, or those who do not track fertility signs daily and meticulously according to guidelines.

The Temperature Method

The temperature method is used by tracking temperature every day at the same time, before talking, eating, drinking, or even getting out of bed. Body temperature changes slightly throughout the menstrual cycle and its fluctuation can help predict ovulation. Temperature is lower in the first part of the cycle and then rises slightly with ovulation. When taken over time, individuals can learn to predict when ovulation will occur. This information can be used to plan when intercourse is more likely to result in pregnancy. (Intercourse right around ovulation is most likely to result in pregnancy.)

The Cervical Mucus Method

The cervical mucus method uses changes in consistency of cervical mucus to predict ovulation and therefore fertility. The mucus on the cervix of the uterus changes in color and consistency during different stages of the menstrual cycle. By reaching into the vaginal canal and obtaining cervical mucus, wiping the vaginal opening with clean toilet paper before urinating, or looking at discharge on underwear, a woman can examine and make a note of the color and texture of her cervical mucus. Just after menstruation, cervical mucus is usually absent, and these are considered "dry days." As the egg begins to ripen, mucus is typically cloudy and white and will feel sticky. Right before ovulation, mucus feels slippery like raw egg whites and can be stretched between fingers. These days are considered "slippery days" and are the days that sex is most likely to result in pregnancy. After several days of that texture and color, the mucus will become cloudier and then will go to dry days again before bleeding begins and the cycle repeats. Tracking the cycle will help to predict timing of ovulation as well. This method is often used in addition to other methods.

The presence of infections, hormonal birth control, breastfeeding, douching, and procedures on the cervix may all impact cervical mucus and make this method less effective.

The Calendar Method

The calendar method estimates fertility by tracking the menstrual cycle over at least six periods. This is done by making a note of the first day of the menstrual period and then the first day of next period. Then count the number of days between cycles. This is then done with six cycles.

Then, take the shortest cycle number (i.e. twenty-seven days) and subtract eighteen from that number (i.e. 27-18=9). Then count that number from the first day of the current cycle and mark that day with an *x* or other notation. The day marked with an *x* is the first fertile day.

Next, find your last fertile day. To do that, find the longest cycle on record and subtract eleven from the number of days in that cycle (i.e. 31-11=20). Count that number from day one of your current cycle, and then mark that day with an x. The day marked with an x is your last fertile day.

This method is less effective with irregular menstrual cycles and should not be used if all cycles are shorter than twenty-seven days.

Lactational Amenorrhea Method (LAM) (Breastfeeding as Birth Control)

Lactational Amenorrhea is when ovulation stops while breastfeeding. Those who rely on this as a form of birth control use exclusive breastfeeding for up to six months to reduce the risk of becoming pregnant. This means breastfeeding "on demand" at least every four hours during the day and at least every six during the night without any supplemental feeding (water, formula, food). New mothers can typically use this effectively if menstrual bleeding has not returned after two months post-partum, the body is fed "on demand" with criteria outlined above, and the baby is less than six months old.

Out of a hundred women who use LAM during the first six months following childbirth, one to two of them may become pregnant.

Other Methods

Abstinence and "Outercourse"

Abstinence from heterosexual intercourse is the only 100 percent effective method to avoid pregnancy. Some people may choose to avoid penis-in-vagina sex for a multitude of reasons and may instead explore sexuality through other activities. "Outercourse" can mean lots of different things to different people. To some it may mean doing everything but penile-vaginal penetration (including fingers, toys, oral sex, and anal sex), and for others it may mean no penetration at all. Some may consider outercourse to mean just kissing, massage, "dry humping," and masturbation.

The chance of getting pregnant from doing "outercourse" is rare but not impossible and varies considerably depending on the activity. For example, anal sex performed on a female that results in male ejaculation could result in pregnancy, as semen can easily enter the vagina if ejaculation occurs near it. Additionally, if a woman is manually penetrated by someone who has semen on their fingers or by a sex toy with semen on it, pregnancy could potentially occur. Sperm can live outside the body for a short time and can likely survive longer on surfaces that are warm and wet.

Withdrawal ("Pulling Out")

Withdrawal is used as a form of birth control when the penis is removed from the vagina just prior to ejaculation. Using this method effectively can be challenging for a variety of reasons, particularly among those who are not sexually experienced.

Pulling out takes a lot of self-control and body awareness. Men who are good at this method can read their sexual responses well and accurately predict when ejaculation is about to occur. Another barrier is that, prior to ejaculation, pre-ejaculatory fluid is released. This fluid may contain sperm and many men are not able to tell when this is occurring. Men must also pull out completely, and ejaculate far enough from the vulva that no sperm reaches it.

As they say, this method is "better than nothing," though far from the most effective way to prevent pregnancy. Used alone it does not provide protection against many STIs. Its efficacy can be enhanced by combining it with other forms of birth control.

Permanent Birth Control Methods

Tubal Ligation

Tubal ligation is a permanent form of birth control which involves making a small abdominal incision to reach the fallopian tubes in females, and then blocking and/or removing a portion of the tubes before tying and sealing them. This prevents sperm from reaching the eggs, therefore preventing fertilization. It is intended to be a permanent form of birth control.

Transcervical Sterilization Procedure (Brand Name Essure)

When using transcervical sterilization for permanent birth control, a trained medical provider inserts a flexible insert through the vagina-cervix-uterus into the fallopian tubes. For the three months following insertion, scar tissue forms in order to block semen from reaching eggs during ovulation. It is intended to be a permanent form of birth control.

Vasectomy

This procedure is performed on males and involves making a small incision on each side of the scrotum in order to reach the vas deferens. The vas deferens are then cut and tied. It does not affect sexual functioning or ejaculation, but simply keeps sperm cells from entering the semen. It is intended to be a permanent form of birth control.

CHAPTER TEN

....

Developing Healthy Relationships

Knowing the Difference Between the Good and the Bad

Cultivating relationships with other people may be one of life's greatest gifts. Being able to successfully nurture relationships can have many benefits, including improving the health of young people and adults. A longitudinal study out of Harvard University followed students from 1938 over almost eighty years and found that positive relationships helped people live longer, healthier, and happier lives.[50] The study indicated that close relationships are even more powerful than money or fame at keeping people happy throughout their lives. It revealed that strong social ties protect people from the upsetting things that happen in life and help to delay the mental and physical declines that accompany aging. Strong social bonds can impact the immune system and cardiovascular system, help us sleep better, and have benefits for our cognitive health. The same study found that close relationships are even better predictors of long and happy lives than are genetics, IQ, and social class.

Relationships can make us feel good and help us to learn cooperation, reciprocity, and other important skills that can provide benefits in nearly every aspect of life.

Learning what a healthy relationship looks and feels like from a young age sets the foundation for future friendships and romantic relationships. Learning to identify and contrast the characteristics of healthy and unhealthy relationships can help all of us to get the most from our partnerships and reduce or eliminate relationships that do not serve us. Parents play an important role in modeling and encouraging healthy relationships.

It's also important to keep in mind that kids' relationships and interactions today likely look different from the relationships that we all remember from our childhood. Kids spend countless hours side by side or through their headsets playing video games. Young people interact twenty-four seven through texting and social media, through images and brief written communication. Conversations, arguments, and misunderstanding can escalate and be mass-distributed throughout entire friend groups in less than a second with the simple act of pressing "send." And among teens who have dating experience, 24 percent of them dated or hooked up with the person that they had met first online, according to Pew Center research.[51] Youth today have little "downtime" when they cannot be contacted by both those with whom they have positive and negative relationships. They have less practice resolving conflict face to face and with verbal interaction through phone conversations. And when relationships are unhealthy, the negative interactions can come from all angles—text, Facebook, twitter, phone, and other channels. Navigating modern friendships among young people likely looks vastly different in many ways, yet those relationships are still just as important.

To add to the unique challenges of navigating modern relationships, the age of the onset of puberty has fallen with progressive generations in many developed countries. People are entering puberty and developing sexually at younger and younger ages, adding new challenges that come with being "romantically interested" in others at younger ages. Social environments for children have also changed in other ways as well, including a greater likelihood of father absenteeism in the home, higher levels of divorce, and the greater likelihood of being raised in blended families. Kids additionally are faced with a number of conflicting images of relationships. On one hand, they are raised with a new level of constant media exposure coupled with a Disney version of *marriage and happily ever after* that they are forced to contrast with the realities of real-life relationships. This generation also has the unique ability to create doctored images of themselves and their social experiences on social media, creating an even more intense gap between what "should be" and what "actually is." Youth growing up in a post #MeToo society are also exposed to the many examples of sexual harassment that saturate the media and perpetrators even among their heroes, which possibly even threatens to normalize and desensitize them to its impacts.

Just as healthy relationships have many benefits, unsatisfying, unhealthy, and violent relationships can have many negative consequences. According to the Centers for Disease Control and Prevention (CDC), 9 percent of high school students reported that they had been purposely physically hurt by a dating partner in the past year.[52] Psychological abuse occurs at even higher rates in adolescents, with approximately 20 percent of heterosexual students, and 29 percent of LGBTQ+ students reporting having been psychologically abused by a partner.

Teen dating violence (TDV) can include physical violence, sexual violence, psychological abuse, and stalking. It can also include electronic abuse, with repeated texting and posting of sexual pictures of a partner without the person's consent. According to the recent data from the Youth Risk Behavior Surveillance System (YRBS), one in five female and one in ten male high school youth were physically and/or sexually victimized by a dating partner in the last year.[53]

Unhealthy or violent relationships can have both short- and long-term serious impacts on developing young people. According to the CDC, victims of TDV are more likely to experience symptoms of depression and anxiety, engage in unhealthy behaviors like tobacco, drug and alcohol use, and think about suicide. TDV also sets the stage for problems in future relationships including intimate partner violence (IPV/SV).

Special Populations at Risk for TDV and Sexual Abuse

Teens Who Identify as LGBTQ+

In addition to the challenges of adolescence described above, some children have an increased risk of physical and sexual violence. According to the recent YRBS, 23 percent of surveyed students who identified as lesbian, gay, or bisexual (LGB) and had dated someone within the last twelve months had experienced dating violence, with 18 percent of LGB students reporting having been forced to have sexual intercourse at some point in their lives.[54] Additionally, LGB teens are more likely than heterosexual youth to experience bullying, physical violence, and rejection. The ways in which parents engage with their children who identify as LGBTQ+ can have a significant impact on their relationships and current and future mental and physical health.

Parents can show support and foster healthy behaviors and relationships in the following ways:

- Find ways to show your teen that they are valued. Continue to include your teen in family events and activities. LGBTQ+ teens who report feeling valued by their parents are less likely to experience depression, attempt suicide, use drugs and alcohol, and become infected with a sexually transmitted disease. In contrast, teens who report parental rejection are more likely to experience each.

- Talk and listen in a way that encourages open discussion about sexual orientation and how to avoid risky behaviors and unsafe situations.

- Stay involved in your child's life and activities. Know who their friends and romantic partners are and make a consistent effort to convey that you care and want them to be safe.

- Support can be expressed through open and honest conversations about problems and concerns. Monitor for behaviors that may indicate that a teen is a victim of violence or drug abuse and victimizing others.

- If suspecting bullying, violence, or depression, take immediate action by seeking out professional help and working with school personnel.

- Build a positive relationship with a teen's teachers and school personnel.

- Help your child find appropriate organizations that cater to the needs of LGBTQ+ youth so that they can establish a peer support system.

Resources

- Centers for Disease Control and Prevention: Lesbian, Gay, Bisexual and Transgender Health

- www.cdc.gov/lgbthealth/youth.htm

- Parental Monitoring

- https://www.cdc.gov/healthyyouth/protective/pdf/parental_monitoring_factsheet.pdf

- Advocates for Youth

- www.advocatesforyouth.org/parents-sex-ed-center-home

- American Psychological Association

- www.apa.org/topics/sexuality/orientation.aspx

- Family Acceptance Project

- familyproject.sfsu.edu

- Gender Spectrum Education and Training

- www.genderspectrum.org

- Parents, Families and Friends of Lesbians and Gays (PFLAG)

- www.pflag.org

Intellectual and Physical Disabilities

People with intellectual and physical disabilities are at an increased risk of experiencing rape and sexual assault. Consent is an important part of healthy sexual activity and can be even more critical and complex when applied to individuals with disabilities. People with disabilities may not have the same access to sexuality education and information about consent. Depending on the disability, it may not be possible for the person to give consent for sexual activity. Some of the factors that may place people with disabilities at an increased risk according to RAINN include:[55]

- An inability to communicate effectively.

- Possessing a general feeling of powerlessness.

- Having a lack of experiential knowledge.

- Living in a hyper-controlled environment.

- Requiring regular assistance from a person who is abusing them and relying on them for access to tools like a computer or phone. The perpetrators may use that power to threaten, coerce, or force a person into nonconsensual sex or sexual activity.

- Possessing a limited ability to access communication tools for reporting.

- Having a lack of information or understanding about healthy sexuality and appropriate touching. This is exacerbated if the person's disability rrequires other people to touch them while providing care.

According to RAINN, parents and other caretakers can reduce the risk of sexual assault among those with disabilities in the following ways:

- Engage—Consistently and effectively communicate with individuals with disabilities about behaviors that are acceptable and not acceptable using straightforward and specific language using examples.

◊   "It is ok for someone to help you dress, but if you feel uncomfortable or they touch your breasts or genitals—that is not ok, and you can tell XYZ immediately."

- Make reporting accessible—Provide information on websites and other sources that link to law enforcement or other reporting outlets. The more access and opportunities an individual has to report, the more likely it will be that they do.

- Educate—Increase access to information about sexual assault and abuse in school curricula and other community spaces. Work to educate law enforcement and care providers and others who may interact with individuals with disabilities about how to respond to a disclosure of assault or abuse.

- Screen caretakers by contacting multiple references that can vouch for their ability, past interactions, and character.

- Seek background checks for caregivers. Also run a search on the National Sex Offender Public Website which pulls data from state, territory, and tribal sex offender registries.

- Do a google search of the caregivers. Look for any red flags. Check social media sites for any information that may cause concern.

- Drop in unannounced on care sessions.

If you believe someone with a disability is or has been the victim of sexual assault, you can report it by calling your local police station or 911. If the person being abused is considered a vulnerable adult under your state laws, you may also be able to contact the local Department of Human Services or Department of Social Services.

If you or the person reporting is deaf, reach out via video phone 1.855.812.1001

To speak with someone who is trained to help, call the National Sexual Assault Hotline at 800.656.HOPE (4673) to be connected with your local sexual assault service provider.

You can chat online anonymously with a support specialist trained by RAINN at online.rainn.org.

Other resources for survivors with disabilities include:

CAVANET: This organization addresses violence against women, human rights, genocide, and crime victims with disabilities.

National Disability Rights Network: NDRN members investigate reports of abuse and neglect, seek systemic change to prevent further incidents, advocate for basic rights, and ensure accountability in health care, education, employment, housing, transportation, and within the juvenile and criminal justice systems for individuals with disabilities.

To speak with someone who is trained to help, call the National Sexual Assault Hotline at 800.656.HOPE (4673) or chat online at online.rainn.org.

Developing healthy, close relationships (including romantic relationships) during adolescence is important and can help young people develop social skills and grow emotionally. It can also help young people transfer these skills to other settings, including relationships with employers, teachers, and even family members. It is normal for young people to pursue relationships and about 35 percent of teens ages thirteen to seventeen have some experience with dating and romantic relationships. It is also normal not to date, with about two-thirds of teens ages thirteen to seventeen reporting not having experience with dating or a romantic relationships, according to recent data from the Pew Research Center.[56] Since dating relationships begin in early adolescence, prevention approaches ideally start young in order to be effective in deterring teen dating violence. Cultivating healthy relationships and preventing dating violence should also include many partners, including policy makers, community groups, faith groups, schools, youth accountability, and parents.

Parents and guardians play a crucial role in helping young people to develop healthy relationships and prevent dating violence. One way to help kids to grow into healthy adults is to encourage them to identify the characteristics of healthy relationships, teach them how to spot when relationships aren't healthy, and help them to create a toolbox of strategies to terminate unhealthy relationships and seek help when necessary. Starting early with healthy parent-child relationships and creating positive family dynamics, modeling effective nonviolent communication and conflict resolution skills, and demonstrating nurturing positive interactions based on respect and trust can set young people up for healthy relationships in adolescence. Nurturing positive, healthy teen dating and friendships can result in improved school performance and leadership skills, a more positive self-image, reduced antisocial and unhealthy behaviors, better interpersonal and negotiation skills, and a greater sense of empathy. Establishing those foundations during early childhood, adolescence, and the teen years can foster healthy adult relationships.

Characteristics of healthy relationships are described below and are compiled from a variety of evidence-based sources including the Department of Health and Human Services, the YWCA, the Domestic Abuse Intervention Project, and are adapted from other best practices in violence prevention.[57,58,59] These examples apply generally to relationships for people at a variety of life stages, though some individual examples may not apply to all ages. Children can benefit greatly from seeing these strategies modeled by parents and others in their lives as well as learning to display them in their own relationships.

Characteristics of Healthy Relationships

- Mutual respect—Partners in healthy relationships listen and respond accordingly when the other person is not comfortable doing something and back off without pushing or coercing. Partners respect one another's values. They observe their own and each other's boundaries. Healthy partners are proud of each other and treat the other with kindness. Healthy partners have a friendship.

- Trust—Partners in healthy relationships spend time together and apart and feel ok with that. Some insecurities are normal, but healthy relationships are secure and don't require "checking" behaviors like following them, looking through each other's phones, social media message boxes, or other private belongings.

- Individuality—Each partner has their own hobbies, interests, and friendships. Healthy partners encourage and support friendships outside of their relationship.

- Self-confidence—Healthy partners have an individual sense of confidence in themselves and their partner. They are calm in each other's presence and can express individual opinions even if not mutually agreed upon.

- Honesty—In healthy partnerships, people feel like they can safely tell the truth and do. They talk openly about feelings even if the topics are difficult. Healthy partners admit when they are wrong and hold themselves accountable.

- Shared responsibility—Healthy relationships involve mutual contribution, both to the relationship itself as well as tasks associated with the partnership. There is a fair distribution of work that is agreed upon by the partners. Decisions are made together.

- Nonthreatening behavior—Partners in healthy relationships feel safe and comfortable expressing themselves without the threat of retaliation.

- Communication and conflict resolution—Some conflict is normal and healthy. Healthy partnerships involve mutually satisfying resolution to conflict. In healthy relationships, people compromise when possible and consider many factors when addressing conflict. In healthy partnerships, people don't ask their partners to compromise beliefs and morals. Healthy partners can agree to disagree when reaching minor impasses and can move on without harboring resentment.

- Economic partnership—In healthy relationships, decisions involving money are made together and benefit both partners with equity.

- Healthy physical connection—Healthy partners share a physical relationship that they are both comfortable with. Both partners feel that their physical contact matches their values and neither feels pressured to engage in activity outside of their comfort zone.

- Nonviolence—There is no violence in healthy relationships.

Characteristics of Unhealthy Relationships

- Dishonesty—One or both partners keep information from each other or misrepresent the truth. A partner may steal from the other or other people in their lives.

- Dependence—A partner relies exclusively on the other for fulfillment. One or both partners do not have friends or interests outside the relationship. A partner threatens that they "cannot live" without the other and may use that to keep the other from leaving.

- Control—One or both partners dictate what friends the other can have, what they can wear, or how they spend their time. They try to isolate the other from their family and friends through manipulation or threats.

- Hostility—One partner antagonizes the other and misdirects life's frustrations on them. Partners bring up unrelated topics in order to pick fights and create conflict.

- Disrespect—One partner makes fun of the other's interests or destroys things that are important to them. They make disparaging or humiliating comments about the other in private and around others.

- Intimidation—One partners attempts to control the behavior of the other by threatening them with a breakup or other consequences and creating an environment of fear.

- Physical abuse—A partner hits, chokes, pushes, breaks things, or blocks the door when the other tries to leave. It can be physical abuse even it doesn't leave a mark.

- Verbal abuse—A partner calls the other names, insults their appearance, and belittles.

- Emotional abuse—One partner is emotionally manipulative. They may tell the other that they don't deserve love or that nobody else would want them. The partner uses gaslighting to blame the other partner for their anger, abuse, or mistreatment. They may try to make the other believe things about themselves or their friends and family that are untrue.

- Digital abuse—One partner hacks into the other's accounts, controls their social media, or stalks their profiles. They may dictate rules about the who the other can be friends with or what they can post to social media.

- Peer pressure—One partner pressures the other to use drugs, alcohol, or participate in other behaviors that are unhealthy or unwanted.

- Sexual violence—One partner forces or pressures the other to engage in sexual activity that is unwanted or coerced. The partner may stop the other from using birth control or condoms or pressure the other into risky or unwanted sexual situations.

Sexual Violence

According to RAINN, an American is sexually assaulted every seventy-three seconds.[60] There are many types of sexual violence that are defined differently according to where a person lives. These include rape, child sexual abuse, intimate partner sexual violence, and other forms of violence. Sexual violence can have serious psychological, emotional, and physical effects on the people who experience it. Each state varies in terms of age and ability to provide consent to sexual activity. There are also differences in how crimes are punished and in statutes of limitations dependent on state laws. To find out specific laws related to sexual assault in your state, access the following website: www.rainn.org/about-sexual-assault.

Tips for Talking to Kids about Relationships

Engaging in conversations with kids about friendships and other relationships can help to facilitate healthy relationships. Some recommendations for the content of those conversations are described below.

- Ask your kids what they would not do for a friend or to maintain a friendship.

- Ask your kids what would be a "deal breaker" that would cause them to end a friendship or romantic relationship. Have them clarify their boundaries.

- Ask your kids to identify things that people do that demonstrate "not being a good friend" and "being a good friend." Make observations about the same when you spot examples of each.

- Use role play as a strategy for practicing confrontations. This may help kids to practice and gain efficacy when approaching conversations and conflict resolution that might be difficult. When appropriate, resist the urge to "helicopter parent" and instead help them to develop personal potency.

- If you have concerns about your child's friendships or the way they are treated by their friends, wait until you are alone to discuss them. Confronting people publicly, whether they are young or old, can activate defense mechanisms and make the conversations less effective.

- Encourage kids of all ages to apologize when it is appropriate in order to foster accountability in relationships. This also establishes standards for respect in relationships.

- Ask kids how they feel when they are with particular friends. Encourage them to use "feeling" words (safe, judged, nervous, loved, etc.).

- Talk to your child about expectations regarding communication on social media, text, YouTube, and the internet. Clarify your boundaries regarding sending photos, when they should ask for permission before sending information or photos, posting personal information, etc.

- Let your child know that they will never be in trouble for telling you about being inappropriately touched, even if someone tries to manipulate or threaten them to say that they will. People who abuse young people often use those types of threats to keep kids from seeking help.

Ending Relationships

Without getting too existential, and for better or worse, all relationships as they exist on earth are finite and will eventually end. We never know if they will last for days, months, years, or a lifetime. Young people will have many people come in and out of their lives, sometimes by their own choice and sometimes because of circumstances outside of their control. Learning how to end relationships and how to deal with others ending relationships is a necessary part of maintaining good mental and emotional health. With time and change, it sometimes makes sense to end some relationships. Young people may be particularly vulnerable to the hurt that comes along with this loss due to the hormonal and developmental factors that influence adolescence. Parents can be influential by helping young people end relationships and deal with breakups in ways that are healthy.

People respond to loss and the end of relationships in a variety of ways that are all "normal." Some people may feel intense feelings of loneliness and grief, while others may feel a sense of relief, or even a mixture of the two. People may experience feelings of guilt after a breakup or may feel responsible for the sadness in the other person. Anger or feelings of rejection and embarrassment are also common reactions. Sometimes these feelings are expressed as outward emotions, and sometimes these feelings are turned inward and expressed as depression and self-deprecation. Some people work quickly to fill the sense of loss with another person or activity, and others will avoid relationships and activity for a while. As much as we want to shelter others, especially our children, from pain, experiencing this grief is an important part of maturing and allows people to move on more successfully to other relationships. The healing process just takes time.

As a parent, stating the above can be helpful to normalize the grieving process. It can be also just be helpful to sit and listen and let your child know that you are there when they are ready to talk. Validating their emotions is a good way to be supportive. It may feel tempting to minimize their experience but try to avoid that. Showing empathy by saying things like, "I know this is hard" or "Ending relationships is really sad" can be helpful and supportive.

Statements like, "Young love usually doesn't work out" or "She wasn't good for you anyway" are generally not helpful and can make the young person feel belittled in addition to the loss they are experiencing.

You can also show support during breakups by avoiding trying to talk them out of their decision because it was a person that you liked. Even if it is a mistake, making mistakes and navigating the consequences is part of maturing. And if you are happy because you didn't like the person, keep your personal feelings aside as much as possible. Your child will be more likely to open up if they don't feel like they need to defend their decisions or the other person. As a parent, be prepared for the rollercoaster of emotions that your child may experience following loss. Know that there will good and bad days and moments. It may be some time of big mood swings before things begin to level out.

Some other strategies that may be helpful to recommend to those dealing with the loss of a relationship include:

- Taking a break from social media—Social media can sometimes give the appearance that everyone is in healthy, fun relationships. Disengaging from social media for a bit can also allow for healing that may not happen as quickly if people are exposed to pictures and posts from their ex.

- Keeping normal routines—Keeping up with hobbies, schoolwork, sports, and regular sleeping habits can expedite the healing process and limit other losses that may occur as a result of disengaging. This may take a bit to restore.

- Finding ways to maintain self-image—Maintaining one's personal appearance can help with countering some of the impacts of breakups. Finding ways to engage in activities that make the person feel competent and accomplished can be helpful to counteract the temporary blow to self-esteem that sometimes comes with breakups.

- Cut off all contact, at least temporarily—Calling, texting, meeting up to talk can extend the grieving process and make breakups more difficult. Physical and virtual space can allow a person to process the breakup and can often give room for clarity that isn't possible when contact is still occurring.

- Stay active—Physical activity can provide a natural enhancement in mood as well as provide many other benefits for emotional and physical health.

- Be selective about confidants—Finding people to talk to and connect with is an important part of the healing process. But avoid talking about the breakup to people who escalate and elevate feelings of anger or despair. Vent to people who will listen without shame, judgement, or escalation.

- Talk to a therapist—If feelings of despair or anger make someone feel as though they will hurt another or themselves, it may be helpful to seek help from a counselor. If the person cannot get out of bed, is missing school or work, is eating a lot less or more, is feeling hopeless about the future, or is using drugs or alcohol to numb the pain, working with a trained mental health care provider may be beneficial.

CHAPTER ELEVEN

··

Talking to Kids about Sex

The "What's," the "How's," and the "When's" of Sex-Positive Parenting

Though many different definitions exist for the phrase "sex positive" as used in this text, the goal of sex-positive parenting is to help children to grow into autonomous, healthy, sexually active adults with positive relationships. Sex-positive parenting, as described here, is about protecting and empowering young people. Parental conversations about sexuality can be very powerful and can result in delayed sexual initiation and increased birth control use and condom use, according to the National Survey of Family Growth.[61]

Sex-positive parenting:

- Normalizes body functions

- Models shame-free discussion about sex, including sexual activity beyond only penile-vaginal sex

- Recognizes that sexual orientation and gender identity are nonbinary

- Focuses on feeling prepared vs. scared

- Teaches consent as a life skill

- Emphasizes the difference between touching that is safe and unsafe

- Directs conversations about sexually transmitted infections toward facts and not fear tactics

- Uses correct terminology when discussing body parts and sexual identities

- Is open to all kids about menstruation and normalizes menstrual health

- Is focused on informed prevention including condom use and pregnancy prevention

- Emphasizes the limitations and potentially problematic impacts associated with the construct of "virginity"

- Normalizes masturbation and pleasure as a normal part of maturation and personal exploration

- Is honest about sexual pleasure and emphasizes both the benefits of sexual relationships along with the risks that accompany them.

The content of the sexuality-education curriculum that children are exposed to at school varies greatly by country and by state. Some of the most notable differences between curricula include the age at which instruction begins, the inclusion or absence of medically accurate materials, the inclusion or absence of information about healthy relationships and consent, the inclusion or absence of content on birth control options, the inclusion or absence of topics related to sexual identity and LGBTQ+ inclusion, and the inclusion or absence of content related to sexual assault prevention and dating violence.

Parents can be effective partners in the sexuality education of their children. Kids receive "sex education" every day. Every time they hear about a public figure touching someone without their consent, or hear about sexual assault on the news, or hear music with sexually suggestive lyrics, or sit in a classroom and hear about sexual development, they are receiving "sex education." Though parents likely have little control over school curriculum or other exposure to "sex education," they do have control over conversations that happen at home.

The following recommendations are adapted from several sources (listed below) and serve as a guide to facilitate open, honest, age-appropriate conversations with your child regarding a variety of topics related to sex and relationships. Each grouping will include a list of things that children should know and understand within those age categories. Hopefully, children will also be learning about these things in school and your role will be to serve as an additional resource. Some kids find it comforting to be able to ask questions at home that they are not comfortable asking at school. Some kids may not be exposed to any of this content in school and will rely heavily on you and other sources for this information. In my years of teaching these topics, I have certainly found that there is a very wide range in knowledge among young people about sexuality, even those who come from the same school districts.

It is ideal to start discussing sexuality when kids are young, which will make the conversations easier and more natural over time. But if your kids are older, it's not too late! You may want to also review the topics suggested for younger children and play a little "catch up" if it is appropriate.

This list is intended to be a *resource* and not a *prescription*. You aren't expected to be a sex ed expert. Many of the suggestions recommend locating outside resources that can be helpful if any of the questions feel outside of your comfort level. Discuss what feels appropriate to you. The list of topics can feel daunting at first glance. Remember that many of these topics may also be discussed at school, and that you are *one partner* in your child's sexuality education. This guide should help you to be a more effective partner, regardless of how much of it you choose to use. Every child is different, and you will likely have a good sense of their maturity level and their readiness to process information related to sexually. The suggestions are designed to be research-based, to facilitate healthy sexual development and personal safety, but should also be adapted as necessary and appropriate.

Suggested topics described below were compiled using modified recommendations based on information from many evidence-based sources including the CDC's Health Education Curriculum Analysis Tool (HECAT),

Guidelines for Comprehensive Sexuality Education: Kindergarten through Twelfth Grade, and *Consent: The New Rules of Sex Education, Lang, MD.*[62,63,64]

Early Childhood to around Age Five

- Ask children if they would like cuddle or be tickled or to kiss or hug relatives, instead of forcing them to do so. Respect their wishes and levels of comfort when it comes to physical contact. Stop tickling them if they ask you to stop to reinforce boundaries and temporal components of consent. Discuss these boundaries with family and friends as well.

- Teach children to ask permission before hugging or kissing friends. When the answer is no, reinforce that it is ok, and suggest an alternate behavior like waving goodbye. Teach phrases like, "is it ok if I _____?" It is recommended that children ask for consent any time they touch someone else. This adds an extra step to their thought process and reinforces the concept of consent.

- When hitting occurs, use it as an opportunity to foster empathy. Using statements like, "I know you wanted Johnnie to play with you, but when you hit him it made him sad. We don't want Johnnie to be sad because you hurt him."

- Teach kids who to go to if someone is hurt or in trouble. Help them to identify adults who are trustworthy.

- Teach children to help other children when they see that they are hurt and encourage them to talk to trusted adults when they see that.

- Teach children that if someone says no, they are to listen to them and take it seriously. But also teach them to ask permission (asking to play with a friend's toy, asking a friend to move, asking a friend to share).

- Teach children to wash themselves to foster bodily autonomy and independence. This reinforces the concept that individuals have control over what happens to their bodies.

- Use correct terminology to describe genitals, including words like vulva, vagina, penis, testicles, and anus. This will empower children and help them to articulate questions surrounding sexuality. This breaks down stigma and helps to facilitate later conversations. Additionally, slang terms or family-based "coded language" can delay the discovery of sexual abuse and cause dangerous miscommunications to take place.

- Allow children to talk about their bodies and ask questions without being shamed. Teach them to describe feelings and to make observations.

~Ages Five to Eight

- Explain to children that certain people have different levels of access to their bodies. This could include a discussion that, although hugs from mom are ok, hugs from strangers are not.

- Explain that all people, including children, have the right to tell others not to touch their body when they do not want to be touched.

- Teach kids to communicate and articulate their feelings about being touched. Do not force them to hug or hold hands, even to pose for photos. Discuss ways they could respond if someone was touching them in a way that makes them feel uncomfortable.

- Identify parents and other trusted adults they could tell if they were feeling uncomfortable about being touched. Talk about how they could reach out to them.

- Talk about how they could clearly say no if they were in a situation that made them feel unsafe and how to leave an uncomfortable situation.

- Educate children about how their bodies are changing in a way that is positive. Demonstrate your comfort and willingness to engage in conversations about their bodies using proper terminology (including male and female anatomy).

- Help your child to recognize discomfort in other people. Teach them to watch how others respond to them and learn to "check in" to make sure others are ok.

- Talk to your child about what is appropriate when it comes to wearing clothes, nudity, and privacy. Discuss rules for your home and rules in public.

- Discuss hygiene and how to stay clean and healthy.

- Describe how people are the same and different and discuss how to respect people who are different from them.

- Have discussions about how friends, family, media, society and culture influence the ways boys and girls think they should act. Reinforce that every person is different, may not fit "the standards," and is deserving of respect.

- Explain that all living things reproduce.

- Describe different types of families, including families with two moms, two dads, no moms and dads, grandparents, single parents, etc. Identify different kinds of family structures and discuss ways that people can demonstrate respect for different types of families.

- Talk about characteristics that make a friend.

- Identify healthy ways for friends to express feelings to each other.

- Explain what bullying and teasing are and how they can be hurtful. Have your child give examples of what they look like.

- Have your children identify parents and other trusted adults they can tell if they are being bullied or teased and give examples of other ways they could also respond in healthy ways if being bullied or teased.

~Ages Eight to Eleven

- Discuss male and female reproductive systems including body parts and their functions using appropriate medically accurate terminology.

- Explain how the timing of puberty and adolescent development varies considerably and can still be healthy. Many kids experience anxiety about when puberty will happen in comparison with their peers. Ease these concerns and help them to show respect to peers as well.

- Describe the purpose of puberty and how it prepares the body for reproduction.

- Discuss the physical, social, and emotional changes that occur during puberty and adolescence. Brainstorm effective ways your child can manage the emotional highs and lows that come along with puberty and adolescence.

- Describe how friends, family, media, society, and culture can influence ideas about body image. Identify and discuss when you see examples of each.

- Talk about resources for medically accurate information about puberty and personal hygiene. It may be a good idea to give kids a source of information that answers questions that they may be too embarrassed to ask about what to expect from puberty to ease anxiety.

- Have children identify trusted adults that they would feel comfortable talking to about puberty and adolescent health issues.

- Discuss the concept of sexual orientation. Describe the variations that are all "normal," including romantic attraction of an individual to someone of the same gender or a different gender, or other variations of that. Describe also that some people may have little interest or sexual attraction to others, which is also normal.

- Identify parents or other trusted adults of whom students can ask questions about sexual orientation.

- Help children to develop healthy relationship skills by brainstorming ways to treat others with dignity and respect, especially when they are with their peers. Discuss how to show people respect even if they are different from themselves.

- As children start to develop "special friendship" relationships, do not tease them about it. Communicate your expectations clearly about contact and boundaries and ask them open questions to indicate your willingness to be a resource.

- Teach children that within special friendships (and all friendships) it is important to ask permission for physical contact and give examples. "May I hold your hand?" "Is it ok if I kiss you?"

- Describe the process of human reproduction.

- Define HIV and identify some age-appropriate channels of transmission, as well as ways to prevent transmission.

- Discuss the characteristics of healthy relationships. Have children identify healthy characteristics of their friendships and how that makes them feel. Have them describe ways in which they are good friends to others.

- Compare positive and negative ways friends and peers can influence relationships.

- Have children identify other trusted adults they can talk to about relationships. Discuss how they could reach out to them.

- Demonstrate positive ways to communicate differences of opinion while maintaining relationships.

- Talk about teasing, harassment, and bullying and explain why they are wrong. Discuss why people might take part in those behaviors.

- Identify parents and other trusted adults they can tell if they are being teased, harassed, or bullied. Talk about how they would reach out.

- Discuss effective strategies that kids could use to respond when they or someone else are being teased, harassed, or bullied. Discuss how they might also persuade others to take action in ways that are healthy and productive.

- Define sexual harassment and sexual abuse. Identify examples when they present themselves in television, movies, or other sources. Discuss how someone could identify abuse and harassment.

- Have children identify parents or other trusted adults they could tell if they or someone they know was being sexually harassed or abused.

- Have children strategize refusal skills that would be appropriate in various situations (e.g. clear "no" statement, walk away, repeat refusal). Talk about how some strategies may be more effective than others.

~Ages Eleven to Fourteen

- Reinforce expectations about technology, internet, and social media use. This will lay the foundation for later conversations concerning technology-related consent.

- Teach children the importance of reporting. Help them to identify trusted adults and reinforce that if someone touches them in private areas, it is not their fault.

- As children enter middle school, begin to expand discussions of consent to include coercion. Discuss the importance of articulating boundaries and how to handle situations in which someone is trying to persuade them to violate boundaries.

- Begin to discuss sexist and misogynistic narratives. Concepts like "men and boys should be aggressors and girls and women should be submissive" can create misunderstandings. Ask young people what they have heard about these types of scripts and expectations and discuss. Give them opportunities to think more critically about generally accepted social expectations. Movies and television shows can provide good opportunities for critical analysis. Point out situations in which people do not ask for consent and ask questions about how it could have been handled differently.

- Discuss accurate and credible sources of information about sexual health. Describe the difference between evidence-based information and other sources that they may encounter. Describe the limitations that exist in going to peers or the internet to get questions answered.

- Describe the physical, social, cognitive, and emotional changes of adolescence. Talk about the broad range in "normal." Reiterate the importance of showing respect to all different kinds of people during this emotional time.

- Analyze how friends, family, media, society, and culture can influence self-concept and body image. Use television shows, music, and movies as opportunities to critically analyze narratives that can be harmful or positive.

- Identify medically accurate sources of information about puberty, adolescent development, and sexuality and places that children can go to get questions answered that they may be too embarrassed to ask out loud.

- Talk about strategies that might be effective in making important decisions about relationships. Identify peer strategies that seem to be effective and contrast them with strategies that don't work as well. Reflect on strategies that have worked well in other situations.

- Differentiate between gender identity, gender expression, and sexual orientation.

- Talk about external influences that shape one's attitudes about gender, sexual orientation, and gender identity. Discuss ways in which we can demonstrate respect for all people. Talk about the negative consequences of feeling disrespected.

- Discuss sources for accurate information about gender identity, gender expression, and sexual orientation. Identify age-appropriate, medically accurate resources (people, websites, books, etc.) that would be appropriate for learning more.

- Talk about respectful vocabulary related to gender identity, gender expression, and sexual orientation. Describe ways in which people communicate respectfully and disrespectfully about those topics. Talk about ways in which people can communicate respectfully with and about people of all gender identities, gender expressions, and sexual orientations.

- Explain the range of gender roles. Discuss the wide variety in "normal" as it relates to gender roles. Brainstorm how narrowly defined gender roles can be problematic.

- Define sexual intercourse and its relationship to human reproduction. Describe that range of sexual behaviors that carry risk (including same-sex behaviors), even though they may not be defined by some as "sex."

- Discuss sexual abstinence as it relates to pregnancy prevention.

- Examine how alcohol and other substances, friends, family, media, society, and culture influence decisions about engaging in sexual behaviors. Describe the importance of clarifying boundaries and values without the influence of substances or during the "heat of the moment" where decision-making will be more clouded.

- Discuss how one could make use of effective communication skills to support one's decision to abstain from sexual behavior.

- Discuss the health benefits, risks, and effectiveness rates of various methods of contraception, including abstinence and condoms.

- Describe resources that contain medically accurate information about pregnancy prevention and reproductive health care and avoiding sexually transmitted infection.

- Discuss how one could be effective with communication and negotiation skills regarding the use of contraception including abstinence and condoms. Describe examples of communication that may be less effective and contrast.

- Describe what considerations would be necessary in decision-making about sexual activity. Describe the decision-making process and how it could be applied in various situations.

- Discuss the benefits and limitations of using condoms in terms of pregnancy prevention and STI protection. Describe the steps to using a condom correctly and talk about common mistakes and how they can be avoided.

- Define emergency contraception and its use. Identify sources of medically accurate information. Discuss how different methods could be obtained.

- Describe the signs and symptoms of a pregnancy.

- Identify medically accurate sources of pregnancy-related information and support including pregnancy options, safe surrender policies, and prenatal care.

- Talk about how prenatal practices can impact birth outcomes and have long-term consequences. Discuss factors that can contribute to a healthy pregnancy including the benefits of planned pregnancy.

- Discuss STIs, including HIV, and how they are and are not transmitted. Discuss the concept of safe, safer, and unsafe sexual contact. Discuss how sexual activity can be made safer. Compare and contrast behaviors, including abstinence, to determine the potential risk of STI/HIV transmission from each.

- Identify medically accurate sources of information about STIs, including HIV.

- Discuss how alcohol and other drugs can impact safer sexual decision-making and sexual behaviors. Clarify values surrounding substance use.

- Describe the signs, symptoms, and potential impacts of STIs, including HIV.

- Discuss ways in which communication skills could be used to reduce or eliminate risk of STIs, including HIV.

- Encourage your child to develop a plan to eliminate or reduce risk for STIs, including HIV.

- Identify local STI and HIV testing and treatment resources. Discuss how they could be accessed if needed.

- Compare and contrast the characteristics of healthy and unhealthy relationships. Use examples from books, television shows, and movies to practice critical analysis. Discuss how you know when relationships are healthy and unhealthy. Analyze the ways in which friends, family, media, society, and culture can influence relationships.

- Explain the criteria for evaluating the health of a relationship. Strategize communication skills that foster healthy relationships.

- Discuss how some relationships can make people vulnerable. Describe the potential impacts of power differences such as age, disability, status, or position within relationships.

- Analyze the similarities and differences between friendships and romantic relationships.

- Talk about the ways in which people express affection in different types of relationships. Discuss your expectations for their behavior and have your child think about what they view as appropriate for themselves.

- Talk about personal boundaries and communication strategies that would be effective in communicating those boundaries. Talk about how people can show respect for other people's boundaries in a variety of types of relationships.

- Discuss ways in which communicating using technology and social media can be beneficial for relationships and harmful for relationships. Discuss how the negative aspects could be reduced and the positive aspects enhanced. Talk about expectations regarding the use of social media and technology.

- Work with your child to develop a plan to stay safe when using social media. Describe strategies to use social media safely, legally, and respectfully.

- Describe situations and behaviors that constitute bullying, sexual harassment, sexual abuse, sexual assault, incest, rape, and dating violence. Use media including television shows and movies as opportunity to bring up these topics and identify examples.

- Identify sources of support such as parents or other trusted adults that they can go to if they or someone they know are being bullied, harassed, abused, or assaulted. Describe how they could be reached and effective ways to communicate that information.

- Describe ways to treat others with dignity and respect in person and online. Discuss ways that a young person could advocate for safe environments that encourage dignified and respectful treatment of everyone.

- Discuss the impacts of bullying, sexual harassment, sexual abuse, sexual assault, incest, rape, and dating violence and why they are wrong.

- Explain why a person who has been raped or sexually assaulted is not at fault.

~Ages Fourteen to Eighteen

- Teach concept of "FRIES" as it applies to consent (see description in Chapter Four).

- Reinforce the differences between "affirmative and enthusiastic consent" and simply just not saying no. Contemporary examples on the news can create appropriate context for these conversations.

- Reinforce message that consent applies to both males and females. Social cues can often make it difficult for males to come forward if their boundaries have been violated. Explain that consent applies to all people, all genders, and all power differentials.

- Have open conversations about pornography. By opening up conversations about pornography, parents can dismantle some of the misguided expectations that pornography can reinforce. Much of pornography contains "fantasy" scenarios that can be unrealistic and even damaging. In the absence of education, young people may internalize false expectations about what communication, gender roles, sex, and consent should look like.

- Discuss what healthy relationships and communication look like. Point out when you see positive examples. Teaching about consent is much more than assault avoidance and is best approached by framing it with positive expectations about relationships.

- Talk about consent, sexting, and the law. Find out what the laws are in your area and make sure your child is aware as well.

- Mentor teenage and college-aged boys around topics of masculinity. Ask them about healthy ways to express masculinity and ways that are unhealthy or that violate the boundaries of others.

- Talk openly and honestly about partying. Reiterate that alcohol and drug use can compromise the ability of an individual to provide consent as well as compromise a person's ability to read signals that another person may be sending. Make your expectations about their behavior clear. Additionally, ask questions about how people might reduce the risks associated with partying in order to ensure safety. Also, develop a plan to put in place in the case the person finds themselves in a dangerous situation (when a driver has had too much to drink, a person finds themselves around people being unsafe, etc.).

- Describe the human sexual response cycle, including the role hormones play.

- Talk about how brain development can impact the emotions and actions of those in adolescence and adulthood. Describe the impacts of that, both positive and negative. Discuss the social and emotional changes of adolescence and early adulthood.

- Brainstorm decision-making models that might be appropriate when approaching situations related to sexual health.

- Reiterate differences between biological sex, sexual orientation, and gender identity and expression. Continue to analyze the influence of friends, family, media, society, and culture on the expression of gender, sexual orientation, and identity.

- Compare and contrast the advantages and disadvantages of abstinence and other contraceptive methods, including condoms.

- Analyze influences that may have an impact on deciding whether or when to engage in sexual behaviors. Clarify values and expectations surrounding these decisions.

- Describe where young people can go to access medically accurate information about contraceptive methods, including abstinence and condoms.

- Encourage young people to think about ways they can effectively communicate their decisions about whether or when to engage in sexual behaviors. Clarify the importance of establishing these boundaries when thinking clearly and removed from any peer pressure or substance.

- Discuss how to apply a decision-making strategy to choices about contraception, including abstinence and condoms.

- Reiterate the steps to using a condom correctly.

- Revisit discussions about emergency contraception and describe how it works and how to obtain it. Identify sources of medically accurate information.

- Identify the laws related to reproductive and sexual health care services (i.e., contraception, pregnancy options, safe surrender policies, prenatal care) in your state. Communicate that information to your child.

- Describe factors that might influence decisions about pregnancy and childbearing. Discuss where someone could go to get medically accurate information about pregnancy and pregnancy options.

- Describe prenatal practices that can contribute to or threaten a healthy pregnancy. Discuss where someone could go to get medically accurate information about pregnancy and pregnancy options.

- Assess the skills and resources needed to become a parent. Discuss the impact of the absence of those skills and resources.

- Find out about and discuss the laws relating to pregnancy, adoption, abortion, and parenting.

- Describe common symptoms of and treatments for STIs, including HIV. Emphasize that many STIs have no visible symptoms and that you often cannot tell if someone has a sexually transmitted infection just by their appearance.

- Find out where someone could go to access local STI and HIV testing and treatment services and discuss.

- Talk about how someone could effectively communicate with a partner about STI and HIV prevention and testing. Describe why this could be difficult and strategize around navigating these conversations.

- Encourage your child to apply a decision-making model to choices about safer sex practices, including abstinence and condoms.

- Talk about the effectiveness of abstinence, condoms, and other safer sex methods in preventing the spread of STIs, including HIV.

- Analyze factors that could influence condom use and other safer sex decisions. Discuss where your child could access medically accurate information about STIs, including HIV.

- Encourage your child to develop a plan to eliminate or reduce risk for STIs, including HIV. Encourage them to think about how they could advocate for sexually active youth to get STI/HIV testing and treatment.

- Find out the local laws related to sexual health care services, including STI and HIV testing and treatment in your community and communicate them to your child.

- Discuss characteristics of healthy and unhealthy romantic and/or sexual relationships. Use examples from media sources to identify healthy and unhealthy characteristics. Discuss how one could identify if they were in an unhealthy relationship.

- Discuss how media can influence one's beliefs about what constitutes a healthy sexual relationship. Have your child clarify their own values and boundaries as they relate to relationships.

- Discuss how to access valid information and resources to help deal with relationships.

- Discuss effective strategies to avoid or end an unhealthy relationship.

- Discuss the range of ways to express affection within healthy relationships.

- Analyze factors, including alcohol and other substances, that can affect the ability to give or perceive the provision of consent to sexual activity.

- Brainstorm effective ways to communicate personal boundaries as they relate to intimacy and sexual behavior. Discuss how to demonstrate respect for the boundaries of others as they relate to intimacy and sexual behavior.

- Describe ways that people can advocate for safe environments that encourage dignified and respectful treatment of everyone.

- Talk about how to be a good friend to someone who has experienced sexual trauma. Discuss ways to access accurate information and resources for survivors of sexual abuse, incest, rape, sexual harassment, sexual assault, and dating violence.

- Identify ways in which they could respond when someone else is being bullied or harassed.

- Talk about why using tricks, threats, or coercion in relationships is wrong. Discuss examples of what that might look like in friendships and romantic relationships.

- Discuss the external influences and societal messages that impact attitudes about bullying, sexual harassment, sexual abuse, sexual assault, incest, rape, and dating violence.

- Reiterate why a person who has been raped or sexually assaulted is not at fault.

Resources

"I Want to Know More about Sex!"

Amaze

Fun, animated videos for young people ages four to fourteen with information about sex, bodies, and relationships.

amaze.org

Centers for Disease Control and Prevention

This site provides a wealth of data and information on all topics related to health, including information about sexually transmitted infections, birth control, and health recommendations.

www.cdc.gov

The Center for Sexual Pleasure and Health

The CSPH is a sexuality training and education organization that works to reduce sexual shame, challenge misinformation, and advance the field of sexuality by providing training and resources for health care providers, educators, and counselors.

www.thecsph.org

Common Sense Media

This site provides entertainment and technology recommendations for families.

www.commonsensemedia.org

Feminist Women's Health Center

This site contains comprehensive information about birth control, abortion and pregnancy, sexual health, and other issues related to women's health.

www.fwhc.org

Go Ask Alice!

This site offers answers to questions about all things health related and is supported by a team of Columbia University health-promotion specialists, health care providers, and other health professionals, along with a staff of information and research specialists and writers.

www.goaskalice.columbia.edu

Guttmacher Institute

This website provides information about research and policy related to sexual and reproductive health and rights.

www.guttmacher.org

Jensplaining

A blog-like, entertaining show aimed at "mythbusting" many common misperceptions about issues related to female sexual anatomy.

drjengunter.com/tv-show

The Kinsey Institute

This site provides a variety of research findings related to love, sexuality, gender, and sexual health.

kinseyinstitute.org

National Sexuality Education Standards

This document provides guidance on essential, minimum, core content for sexuality education for K–12 in schools.

siecus.org/resources/national-sexuality-education-standards

Office on Sexual Orientation and Gender Diversity

This site provides information about gender identity and sexual orientation pertaining to people who identify as lesbian, gay, bisexual, or transgender.

www.apa.org/pi/lgbt

Parents, Families, Friends, and Allies of Lesbians and Gays

A network to provide opportunity for conversation about sexual orientation and gender identity with a goal of increasing respect for human diversity.

www.pflag.org

Planned Parenthood

This site provides health care provider information and sexuality-education information including comprehensive information about sexually transmitted infections and birth control.

www.plannedparenthood.org

The Rape, Abuse, & Incest National Network (RAINN)

RAINN is an American nonprofit anti-sexual assault organization which operates the National Sexual Assault Hotline, as well as the Department of Defense Safe Helpline, and carries out programs to prevent sexual assault, help survivors, and ensure that perpetrators are brought to justice through victim services, public education, public policy, and consulting services.

www.rainn.org

Scarleteen

Inclusive, comprehensive, supportive sexuality and relationship information for teens and young adults.

www.scarleteen.com

SEICUS: Sex Ed for Social Change

SEICUS develops, collects, and disseminates information, promotes comprehensive education about sexuality, and advocates for the right of individuals to make responsible sexual choices.

siecus.org

Sex, etc.

Resource for honest and accurate sexual health information including terminology, teen's rights, sex education, and more.

sexetc.org/about

Acknowledgements

Thank you to Bailey, who not only allowed me to write about our initial "birds and the bees" talk in my book, but also put up with me being a sex educator at her university. If that isn't worthy of sainthood, I am not sure what is. Thank you also for all the years of tolerating mom being busy and having weird sex books all over the house. Being your mother is the single greatest joy of my life.

Thank you to my mother, who was and is the best role model of selfless parenting I could have ever asked for.

Thank you to all the educators and advocates who tirelessly work to create an empowering, inclusive environment for our young people.

Thank you for those who support science and evidence-based practice. The world needs you.

Lastly, thank you to the Mango Publishing group for believing in this project. Thank you for your support, guidance, and patience.

Endnotes

1   "Teen Pregnancy Rates Declined in Many Countries Between the Mid-1990s and 2011," News Release, Guttmacher Institute, accessed May 5, 2020, www.guttmacher.org/news-release/2015/teen-pregnancy-rates-declined-many-countries-between-mid-1990s-and-2011.

2   "Adolescent fertility rate (births per 1,000 women ages 15–19)," Data Bank Microdata Data Catalog, The World Bank, accessed May 5, 2020, data.worldbank.org/indicator/SP.ADO.TFRT.

3   Amy T. Schalet, "Beyond Abstinence and Risk: A New Paradigm for Adolescent Sexual Health," *Women's Health Issues* 21, no. 3 (May 01, 2011). www.whijournal.com/article/S1049-3867%2811%2900008-9/abstract.

4   "16 Critical Sexual Education Topics," Centers for Disease Control and Prevention, accessed May 5, 2020, pubertycurriculum.com/wp-content/uploads/2017/11/16-Critical-Sexual-Education-Topics-CDC.pdf.

5   John S. Santelli, Leslie M. Kantor, Stephanie A. Grilo, Ilene S. Speizer, Laura D. Lindberg, Jennifer Heitel, Amy T. Schalet, Maureen E. Lyon, Amanda J. Mason-Jones, *et al.* "Abstinence-Only-Until-Marriage: An Updated Review of U.S. Policies and Programs and Their Impact." Journal of Adolescent Health 61 (2017): 273–280. www.jahonline.org/article/S1054-139X%2817%2930260-4/pdf.

6   "International technical guidance on sexuality education: An evidence-informed approach," Sexual and Reproductive Health, UNESCO, accessed May 5, 2020, www.who.int/reproductivehealth/publications/technical-guidance-sexuality-education/en.

7   Ashley M. Fox, Georgia Himmelstein, Hina Khalid (PhD), Elizabeth A. Howell (MD), "Funding for Abstinence-Only Education and Adolescent Pregnancy Prevention: Does State Ideology Affect Outcomes?" *American Journal of Public Health*, (February 06, 2019), ajph.aphapublications.org/doi/abs/10.2105/AJPH.2018.304896.

8   Riley J. Steiner, Ganna Sheremenko, Catherine Lesesne, Patricia J. Dittus, Renee E. Sieving and Kathleen A. Ethier, "Adolescent Connectedness and Adult Health Outcomes," *Pediatrics,* 144, no. 1 (2019), pediatrics. aappublications.org/content/144/1/e20183766.

9   Fox, Himmelstein, Khalid, Howell, "Funding for Abstinence-Only Education and Adolescent Pregnancy Prevention."

10   M.K. Hutchinson, "The Parent-Teen Sexual Risk Communication Scale (PTSRC-III): instrument development and psychometrics." Nursing Research, 56, no.1 (Jan-Feb 2007): 1–8, www.ncbi.nlm.nih.gov/ pubmed/17179868.

11   Janis Wolak, Kimberly Mitchell, David Finkelhor, "Unwanted and Wanted Exposure to Online Pornography in a National Sample of Youth Internet Users" Pediatrics 119, no. 2 (February 2007): 247–257, pediatrics. aappublications.org/content/119/2/247?sso=1&sso_redirect_count=1&nfstat us=401&nftoken=00000000-0000-0000-0000-000000000000&nfstatusdescrip tion=ERROR%3a+No+local+token.

12   "Adolescent Sexual and Reproductive Health in the United States," Fact Sheet, Guttmacher Institute, accessed May 5, 2020, www.guttmacher.org/ fact-sheet/american-teens-sexual-and-reproductive-health#.

13   "Talking to Your Kids About Sexual Assault," RAINN, accessed May 5, 2020. www.rainn.org/articles/talking-your-kids-about-sexual-assault.

14   "The Case for Teaching Kids 'Vagina,' 'Penis,' and 'Vulva'," The Atlantic, accessed May 5, 2020, www.theatlantic.com/health/ archive/2013/04/the-case-for-teaching-kids-vagina-penis-and-vulva/274969.

15   "Interagency statement calls for the elimination of 'virginity-testing'," World Health Organization, accessed May 5, 2020, www.who.int/ reproductivehealth/virginity-testing-elimination/en.

16   W. A. Marshall, J. M. Tanner, "Variations in pattern of pubertal changes in boys," *Archives of Disease in Childhood*, London, June 1969, 45 (239): 13–23.

17   W. A. Marshall, J. M. Tanner, "Variations in pattern of pubertal changes in girls," *Archives of Disease in Childhood*, London, June 1969. 44 (235): 291–303.

18   N. Brix, A. Ernst, L. Lauridsen, E. Parner, H. Støvring, J. Olsen, T. B. Henriksen, C. H. Ramlau-Hansen, "Timing of puberty in boys and girls: A population-based study," *Paediatric and perinatal epidemiology*, January 2019, 33 no.1, 70–78. doi.org/10.1111/ppe.12507.

19   Brix, Ernst, Lauridsen, Parner, Støvring, Olsen, Henriksen, Ramlau-Hansen, "Timing of puberty in boys and girls."

20   "The Kinsey Scale," The Kinsey Institute, accessed May 5, 2020, kinseyinstitute.org/research/publications/kinsey-scale.php.

21   "The Kinsey Scale," The Kinsey Institute.

22   "LGBTQ Youth," US Department of Population Affairs, accessed May 6, 2020, www.hhs.gov/ash/oah/adolescent-development/healthy-relationships/lgbtq/index.html.

23   Kelly, *Sexuality Today* (New York: McGraw Hill, 2014), 365.

24   R. Worthington, H. Savoy, F. Dillon, E. Vernaglia, "Heterosexual Identity Development: A Multidimensional Model of Individual and Social Identity," *The Counseling Psychologist* 30, no. 4 (July 2002): 496–531.

25   V. Cass, "Homosexuality Identity Formation," *Journal of Homosexuality* 4, no. 3 (1979): 219–235.

26   "About Sexual Assault," RAINN, accessed May 6, 2020, www.rainn.org/about-sexual-assault.

27   "What is Sexting," Kids Help Phone, accessed May 6, 2020, kidshelpphone.ca/get-info/what-sexting.

28   "The Common Sense Census: Media Use by Tweens and Teens," Common Sense Media, accessed May 6, 2020, www.commonsensemedia.org/sites/default/files/uploads/research/census_researchreport.pdf.

29   "The Effects of Pornography on Children and Young People,"
Australian Government, Australian Institute of Family Studies, accessed May
6, 2020, aifs.gov.au/sites/default/files/publication-documents/rr_the_effects_
of_pornography_on_children_and_young_people_1.pdf.

30   "The Effects of Pornography on Children and Young People,"
Australian Institute of Family Studies.

31   "Teens, Social Media& Technology 2018," Pew Research Center,
accessed May 6, 2020, www.pewresearch.org/internet/2018/05/31/teens-
social-media-technology-2018.

32   "Theories & Approaches: Sexual Risk and Protective Factors," Resource
Center for Adolescent Pregnancy Prevention, accessed May 6, 2020, recapp.
etr.org/recapp/index.cfm?fuseaction=pages.TheoriesDetail&PageID=338.

33   Call to Action: LGBTQ Youth Need Inclusive Sex Education,"
Advocates for Youth, accessed May 6, 2020, answer.rutgers.edu/file/A%20
Call%20to%20Action%20LGBTQ%20Youth%20Need%20Inclusive%20
Sex%20Education%20FINAL.pdf.

34   "Gay and Bisexual Men's Health," Centers for Disease Control and
Prevention, accessed May 6, 2020, www.cdc.gov/msmhealth/STD.htm.

35   J. Steinke, M. Root-Bowman, S. Estabrook, D. Levine, L. Kantor,
"Meeting the Needs of Sexual and Gender Minority Youth: Formative
Research on Potential Digital Health Interventions," Journal of Adolescent
Health 60, no. 5 (May 2017): 541–548.

36   "Guidelines for Comprehensive Sexuality Education," National
Guidelines Task Force, accessed May 6, 2020, siecus.org/wp-content/
uploads/2018/07/Guidelines-CSE.pdf.

37   S. Baines, E. Emerson, J. Robertson, C. Hatton, "Sexual activity
and sexual health among young adults with and without mild/moderate
intellectual disability," BMC Public Health 18, no. 1 (May 2018): 667.

38   W. Masters, V. Johnson, *Human Sexual Response* (Boston: Little,
Brown, and Company, 1966).

39   "Adolescent and School Health," Sexual Risk Behaviors, Centers for
Disease Control and Prevention, accessed May 6, 2020, www.cdc.gov/
healthyyouth/sexualbehaviors/index.htm.

40   "Youth Risk Behavior Surveillance—United States, 207," Morbidity
and Mortality Weekly Report, Centers for Disease Control and Prevention,
accessed May 6, 2020, www.cdc.gov/healthyyouth/data/yrbs/pdf/2017/
ss6708.pdf.

41   "International Technical Guidance on Sexuality Education: An
Evidence-Informed Approach," United Nations Educational, Scientific and
Cultural Organization (UNESCO), accessed May 6, 2020, unesdoc.unesco.
org/ark:/48223/pf0000260770.

42   "HIV and Youth," Centers for Disease Control and Prevention,
accessed May 6, 2020, www.cdc.gov/hiv/group/age/youth/index.html.

43   "Sexually Transmitted Diseases (STDs): Which STD Tests Should I
Get?" Centers for Disease Control and Prevention, accessed May 6, 2020,
www.cdc.gov/std/prevention/screeningreccs.htm.

44   "Sexually Transmitted Disease Surveillance 2018," Centers for Disease
Control and Prevention, accessed May 6, 2020, www.cdc.gov/std/stats18/
infographic-html.htm.

45   "Diseases and Related Conditions," Centers for Disease Control and
Prevention, accessed on May 6, 2020, www.cdc.gov/std/default.htm.

46   "Prevent Unintended Pregnancy," CDC's 6/18 Initiative: Accelerating
Evidence into Action, Centers for Disease Control and Prevention, accessed
May 6, 2020, www.cdc.gov/sixeighteen/pregnancy.

47   "Birth Control," Planned Parenthood, accessed May 6, 2020, www.
plannedparenthood.org/get-care/our-services/birth-control.

48   "Birth Control Patch," Mayo Clinic, accessed on May 6, 2020, www.
mayoclinic.org/tests-procedures/birth-control-patch/about/pac-20384553.

49   "About Nexplanon," Nexplanon, accessed May 6, 2020, www.nexplanon.com/?utm_source=bing&utm_medium=cpc&utm_campaign=Nexplanon_Brand_BRND_NA_ENGM_EXCT_TEXT_FEMALE&utm_term=nexplanon%20website&utm_content=NEXPLANON%20V2&utm_kxconfid=sgaizzyx0&gclid=CMXI85uCoOkCFcWCfgoddgILUg&gclsrc=ds.

50   "Harvard Second Generation Study," Harvard Study of Development, accessed May 6, 2020, www.adultdevelopmentstudy.org.

51   "Teens, Technology, and Romantic Relationships," Pew Research Center, accessed May 6, 2020, www.pewresearch.org/internet/2015/10/01/teens-technology-and-romantic-relationships.

52   "2011 Youth Risk Behavior Surveillance United States," Centers for Disease Control and Prevention, accessed May 6, 2020, www.cdc.gov/mmwr/pdf/ss/ss6104.pdf.

53   "2011 Youth Risk Behavior Surveillance United States," Centers for Disease Control and Prevention.

54   "Lesbian, Gay, Bisexual, and Transgender Health," Centers for Disease Control and Prevention, accessed May 6, 2020, www.cdc.gov/lgbthealth/youth.htm.

55   "Sexual Abuse of People with Disabilities," Rape, Abuse & Incest National Network (RAINN), accessed May 6, 2020, www.rainn.org/articles/sexual-abuse-people-disabilities.

56   "Teens, Technology, and Romantic Relationships," Pew Research Center, accessed May 6, 2020, www.pewresearch.org/internet/2015/10/01/teens-technology-and-romantic-relationships.

57   "What Healthy Dating and Romantic Relationships Look Like," Health and Human Services, accessed May 6, 2020, www.hhs.gov/ash/oah/adolescent-development/healthy-relationships/dating/what-relationships-look-like/index.html.

58   "Power and Control," YWCA, accessed May 6, 2020, ywcaspokane.org/
programs/help-with-domestic-violence/power-and-control-wheel.

59   "What is the Duluth Model?" Domestic Abuse Intervention Programs,
accessed May 6, 2020, www.theduluthmodel.org/what-is-the-duluth-model.

60   "About Sexual Assault," RAINN, accessed May 6, 2020, www.rainn.org/
about-sexual-assault.

61   "Talking with Your Teens about Sex: Going Beyond 'the Talk,'" Centers
for Disease Control and Prevention, accessed May 6, 2020, www.cdc.gov/
healthyyouth/protective/pdf/talking_teens.pdf.

62   "Health Education Curriculum Analysis Tool (HECAT)," Centers
for Disease Control and Prevention, accessed May 6, 2020, www.cdc.gov/
healthyyouth/HECAT/index.htm.

63   "Guidelines for Comprehensive Sexuality Education," National
Guidelines Task Force, accessed May 6, 2020, siecus.org/wp-content/
uploads/2018/07/Guidelines-CSE.pdf.

64   J. Lang, *Consent: The New Rules of Sex Education: Every Teen's Guide to
Healthy Sexual Relationships* (Althea Press, 2018).

About the Author

Robin Pickering is currently an Associate Professor of Health Sciences specializing in Community Health and serves as the Program Director of Women's and Gender Studies at Whitworth University in Spokane, Washington. Her research interests include women's health issues, health risk behaviors, and issues surrounding sexuality. She also works as a consultant for improving gender equity in workplaces, has served as the Vice Chair of the Board for the Spokane AIDS Network, Program Director of Community Health at Eastern Washington University (EWU), and steering committee member for the EWU Masters in Public Health degree. She currently serves as an advisory board member for the Eastern Washington University Alumni magazine, cabinet member for the Whitworth Office of Diversity, Equity, and Inclusion, as well as a contributor for several local media publications. Dr. Pickering received her PhD in Education with an emphasis on Health and Psychology, a master's degree in Exercise Science and Pedagogy, and a bachelor's degree in Health Promotion and Wellness. She has also served on the board for Early Head Start, The Spokane Birth Outcome Task Force, and on various other committees committed to promoting community health. Robin has worked as a certified Wellness Coach and currently serves as a Personal Development Consultant specializing in Sexual Assault Prevention for athletic organizations.

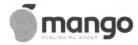

Mango Publishing, established in 2014, publishes an eclectic list of books by diverse authors—both new and established voices—on topics ranging from business, personal growth, women's empowerment, LGBTQ studies, health, and spirituality to history, popular culture, time management, decluttering, lifestyle, mental wellness, aging, and sustainable living. We were recently named 2019 *and* 2020's #1 fastest growing independent publisher by *Publishers Weekly.* Our success is driven by our main goal, which is to publish high quality books that will entertain readers as well as make a positive difference in their lives.

Our readers are our most important resource; we value your input, suggestions, and ideas. We'd love to hear from you—after all, we are publishing books for you!

Please stay in touch with us and follow us at:

Facebook: Mango Publishing
Twitter: @MangoPublishing
Instagram: @MangoPublishing
LinkedIn: Mango Publishing
Pinterest: Mango Publishing

Sign up for our newsletter at www.mangopublishinggroup.com and receive a free book!

Join us on Mango's journey to reinvent publishing, one book at a time.